Life
Begins
at 60!

Advance Praise

"This is an epic book. It's engagingly written and guaranteed to take you further along the road to a happy and fulfilled life. Don't miss it!"

—**Mitzi Perdue** (Mrs. Frank Perdue),
Founder of WinThisFight.org and
author of *52 Tips to Combat Human Trafficking*

"Inspirational! This book personally helps you redraft your life at sixty to be the best 'You' ever."

—**Sue Doane**, Award-Winning Author of
Passion Produces Prosperity

"*Life Begins at 60!* is honest, clever, insightful yet simple and informative. It's a how-to guide on how to live your best life. A must read!"

—**Danielle Stevens**, Executive Assistant at
The Raymond Aaron Group™

"*Life Begins at 60!* is a masterpiece. It helps set women on the path to greatness. I absolutely loved it! It's an awesome read, and I highly recommend it."

—**Alka Sharma**, Alka's Total Fitness Studio Boutique

"*Life Begins at 60!* is a powerful guide to inspire, motivate, and kick-start a new beginning to your life to regain fun, joy, direction, and passion. This incredible book is organized in a way that is easy to read and even easier to follow. Ruth has taken a common problem that affects a lot of women who hit sixty, reflecting on their bodies, careers, health, relationships, sex lives, and more. Your feeling of having a humdrum life will get a new jump-start with simple-to-use ideas and strategies. *Life Begins at 60!* takes the everyday conversations women are having at this stage of their lives and breaks down the key ideas that go through all women's minds—self-confidence, body image, weight, fitness, and more. From there Ruth takes a closer look at a woman's mindset, including self-love, self-talk and accountability, and finally living life without regrets. This is an excellent read for anyone who has come to a place where you need a boost and a reminder that you can make amazing changes for yourself at any age—and you are worth it! You'll find yourself absorbed in the simple yet powerful teachings so many of us forget. We all need and deserve to have a good life. I highly recommend this book for any woman needing guidance for a reset in their lives. It is such a fabulous resource."

—**Brigitte Tritt**, Author, Transformational Therapist and
Certified Life Coach

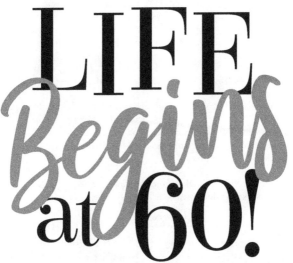

LIFE Begins at 60!

Start Living a Happy Life Full of Purpose

RUTH VERBREE

NEW YORK

LONDON • NASHVILLE • MELBOURNE • VANCOUVER

Life Begins at 60!

Start Living a Happy Life Full of Purpose

© 2021 Ruth Verbree

Published in New York, New York, by Morgan James Publishing. Morgan James is a trademark of Morgan James, LLC. www.MorganJamesPublishing.com

Morgan James BOGO™

A **FREE** ebook edition is available for you or a friend with the purchase of this print book.

CLEARLY SIGN YOUR NAME ABOVE

Instructions to claim your free ebook edition:
1. Visit MorganJamesBOGO.com
2. Sign your name CLEARLY in the space above
3. Complete the form and submit a photo of this entire page
4. You or your friend can download the ebook to your preferred device

ISBN 9781631953972 paperback
ISBN 9781631953989 eBook
Library of Congress Control Number:
 2020949286

Cover Design by:
Rachel Lopez
www.r2cdesign.com

Interior Design by:
Melissa Farr
backporchcreative.myportfolio.com

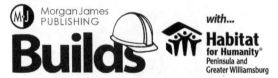

Morgan James is a proud partner of Habitat for Humanity Peninsula and Greater Williamsburg. Partners in building since 2006.

Get involved today! Visit
MorganJamesPublishing.com/giving-back

Contents

Foreword

In youth we learn; in age we understand.
—Unknown

In *Life Begins at 60!* Ruth Verbree has a clear, fresh, and renewed perspective and understanding of life itself. The principles just beyond this page unapologetically highlight some of her most embarrassing mistakes and life's tender moments and, most important, focus on mental successes, emotional advancements, and dismantling physical limitations. *Life Begins at 60!* upends any notion of retirement or the mundane idea of waiting for life to pass by. Ruth Verbree teaches all of us how to restart our lives again no matter what circumstances we may face.

Plenty of books have been written on life lessons, tragedy to triumph, and success, but this one is different. *Life Begins at 60!* is an upbeat approach to help each reader grow through Ruth's transparency in some of her most challenging years of life. Some stories are uncomfortable; yet we know growth happens when we are in the valleys of life, buried in soil and surrounded by darkness. And other discoveries help to reassure, encourage, and motivate each of us to become the best versions of ourselves.

Life Begins at 60! is full of dare and adventure which requires us to commit to greatness, consciously pursue new goals, and stretch ourselves beyond self-sabotaging limits. Some people are comfortable with average, and others avoid living a better life beyond what is considered the norm. But Ruth believes you can become a better person than you were yesterday; that's a good start.

As the daughter of the legendary motivational speaker, Les Brown, in this masterpiece I have gained a renewed focus and jolt of excitement for everyday living. I realize certain areas in my life need a revival. *Life Begins at 60!* reminds me to love myself, accept my flaws, and work on becoming better on a daily basis. The richness, depth, and honesty make *Life Begins at 60!* a true gem of wisdom and priceless insight. I am blessed to have read every page and can only pray I can be like Ruth when I grow up.

Warning: To anyone who finishes this book, a change is bound to occur, and a new life will begin for you right now.

Serena Brown Travis

www.serenabrowntravis.com

Introduction

Dear Holly,

My name is Ruth. We've never met, but I'm a friend of Cara's.

About a year ago she and I got together for lunch and spent hours chatting and connecting over lattes and shared misery. I am sixty years old, and Cara is right on my heels. We couldn't believe how similar our lives had become, and not in ways we appreciated. We had both found ourselves feeling unfulfilled, without purpose, and unhappy. At sixty, we knew it was time to start enjoying life again.

It had been years since we'd seen each other. Casual chit-chat didn't last long, and time seemed to slow down as we fell back into the comfortable rhythm of friendship. It was as if we had never left each other's side. If you have ever had one of those moments with an old friend, you know the kind of elation that comes with it. A sense of relief, safety, and excitement, all at the same time.

Cara and I went deep immediately and soon discovered we were in the same boat. We were both stuck feeling lonely—yes, lonely! Two souls, connected by the past and connected still, both burdened by loneliness—and why? We were both happily married, so to speak . . . but we knew something was missing. We shouldn't have been lonely. We should have been living our best lives by this point! We ought to have been travelling the world, experiencing the things we always dreamed of, loving and laughing all through our sixties.

Neither of us was doing what we wanted to do. Cara was burning herself out, working full-time outside of her home . . . and me? I was working madly to get my entrepreneurial life off the ground. So far, it felt as if all I'd done was spin my wheels and spend my hard-earned retirement money on coaches who were promising me results; only I had yet to see my success.

That was about a year or so ago, and since then so much has changed.

Let me tell you a little bit about who I am. I am an international, award-winning author and speaker, and I have been fortunate to share the stage with megabrand names such as Les Brown, Bob Proctor, Dr. Joe Vitale, Jack Canfield, and many other great speakers. But the best part of my journey has been the ability to help women all over the world realize that life begins at sixty. Together we are finding recipes for joy, beginning and continuing to live a life of bliss rather than living in a world of blah. So here I am, ready to share with you exactly what happened when I met Cara that day and everything that's changed since, all because she made the decision to follow the steps I have taken and incorporate my recipes for joy into her life. Now we are both living life to the fullest, and she and I both know that *Life Begins at 60!*

My question to you is this: What is it you really want to be doing?

I want to help you make your sixties your best years yet. I was like Cara, lonely and blue, overweight, unhappy with life and with myself, until I discovered the blueprint to finding real and lasting joy. Once I discovered this, I realized I wasn't stuck in my misery, and neither are you. Believe it or not, life can truly begin at sixty.

I'm here to show you how.

Over sixty percent of divorces are initiated by women in their menopausal years[1] who are dissatisfied not only with their marriage, but their careers, friendships, sex lives, and the way they look and feel about themselves.

Let me reassure you—if this is you, you're not alone. The very point of this book is that life isn't over for you. There is HOPE. Your passion for life is not lost forever. If you're ready to start living a life of happiness and fulfillment, then you're in the right place.

After experiencing the change in my life and Cara's, I decided to write this book to help women who were also in the same phase of life, because I know how you feel. I have been in your shoes, and I've seen the other side. I want to help you reignite your passion for life as I have.

Our circumstances may be vastly different, but I know our feelings will resonate. My story is honest and real, and I will take you through my ups and downs, the moments of laughter and heartbreak, anger and excitement in my own life. Don't worry—I will not hold back the juicy details, and trust me when I say I have some provocative moments coming up.

I plan to keep you on the edge of your seat as we go through this journey together. I have my own opinions and trust you do as well (we're menopausal women!). But ultimately I have learned experience and wisdom to share with you. You may not want to admit how much my and Cara's stories relate to yours, but I guarantee that as you go through this book you will hear yourself saying things like: "Yes, that's me! I feel the exact same way. I didn't even realize I felt that way!"

This story will inspire you. You will likely laugh, cry, and feel relieved, maybe all at once.

I will share real moments, even the most flirtatious ones, things that most women prefer to keep locked up deep inside themselves. Intimate stories and details will be revealed and come alive instead of being kept secret.

Now does this sound familiar at all? You're exhausted. Burned out! The hot flashes practically kill you, and you've tried everything to hide the wrinkles that keep on getting deeper. You feel sluggish and stuck in a rut; you're sick of living in a cycle that brings no satisfaction. Your life, as you can best describe it, feels totally blah . . . meaningless.

Let's go back in time for a moment. I want you to imagine your wedding day once again. Remember the date and time. (Mine was May 15, 11a.m. That's one date I'll never forget!)

Remember the morning of your wedding day? Remember how you felt when you first awoke. What did you do in those early hours? Probably you were somewhat nervous, excited; you were feeling a rush and a range of emotions. Maybe you felt confident. Maybe you had second thoughts. Regardless of it, the day happened. You went through with the ceremony. Picture that moment . . . that day. Visualize the venue, whether it was a tropical beach or a packed-out church. Did everything go according to plan? Were there funny moments, stressful mishaps? Did everyone make it on time? What do you remember?

Getting ready for your wedding day is an experience like no other. Your hair, makeup, nails, and even the breakfast you ate that day are memories that can't be erased.

Of course, we can't forget the dress. Ohhh, the dress—whether a ballroom gown or a bohemian-style lace dress, you were breathtaking, and you knew it. Take yourself back to that first moment, gazing at yourself in the mirror, ready to walk down the aisle.

Never in your life have so much effort and money gone into one event, but it was worth it. Today you're a princess, and you're about to spend the rest of your life with your Prince Charming. Smile. Remember the joy of it.

Now flash forward to today. Take a look in the mirror. Who do you see now? And what goes through your mind?

"I've changed so much."

"I'm overweight!"

"I look so old."

"I have so many wrinkles."

"I don't look happy."

"I hate my cellulite."

"I wish I still looked like . . . ."

I want to remind you that, deep within, you are still that beautiful young woman! You're in there. In fact, the beauty you hold today carries far more meaning than it did back then. The woman you are now has grown and lived and endured more than that young girl could have dreamed of. You have so much more to give now than ever before. You have more wisdom, more color, more creativity, more compassion, more time, more beauty, more love, and more wrinkles to prove it. There really is a higher calling, a purpose, a mission for your life than the one you feel stuck in right now. Well, this rut is about to end! You are again in the preparation stage for another huge life adventure. You're about to take off, to make a change, to go down the aisle, so get ready to put on your gown! Things will never be the same.

Each step we will take together is like a steppingstone across a river. Think of it like a roadmap to bliss. This guide will take you from wherever you are this moment to a life filled with real joy, a life that begins at sixty (or whatever age you are today).

Before we get started, though, I want to share one more story with you—this is the story of a woman named Josie. At fifty-nine, Josie had been married for almost forty years. Despite a long relationship, she felt miserable, alone, and unhappy in her marriage.

To be frank, Josie had lost her zest for life and for sex. She refused to stay this way and asked her husband to go out dancing with her and hit the town. He said no, but that didn't stop Josie.

She spent all day getting ready (the anticipation was half the fun), got her nails done, and bought a new outfit. She felt confident. She grabbed a girlfriend, and they decided they would have a night of fun on their own.

Before long, they hit the lounge and were dancing the night away. They were making new friends and enjoying the music, and for the first time in a long time Josie felt free and happy. That anticipation, joy, and excitement she remembered from her wedding day reappeared—it was exhilarating.

She suddenly realized she hadn't lost her ability to enjoy life; she had just kept her joy locked up for years, like being in a prison. Josie felt confident and attractive and was approached by different men asking her to dance. She was tempted to indulge, enjoy the moment and get her hormones flowing; but she thought of her husband at home. So she finally left to go home—but she took her renewed desire and mindset with her. You can imagine what transpired that night when she got home . . . a sexual encounter reignited!

After just one amazing night, her passion was back. Now you and I both know there is more to life and feeling purposeful than sex; but for Josie this was the first step to moving forward.

I encourage you to take my invitation to join me and many other women on this journey together. To hear stories of others like you who chose to do so, who have found the kind of life they'd stopped dreaming of.

It's time to change your life, to stop settling, and to experience the greatest happiness life has to offer today. Life really does begin at sixty!

Chapter 1

Decision Time

You Want to Make a Change

The first step in this journey is perhaps the most important, and it's all up to you! Are you sick and tired of feeling sick and tired? Burned out on life, exhausted from simple day-to-day activities, feeling as if you have nothing to live for?

That's exactly where I was. Miserable, lonely—and feeling as if I had no way out.

Picture this: You're at home on a normal day. It's about mid-afternoon when you hear the doorbell ring. You're not expecting anyone; but as you get up to answer the door you glance in the mirror.

Honestly, you're startled by your own appearance. You fight to ignore the thoughts telling you that you look tired and old. You wonder what happened to the woman you used to be. You push the thoughts aside, telling yourself, "It's just a stranger at the door. What does it matter?" You open the door, and, sure enough, you have no idea who is standing in front of you.

"Good morning," you say politely.

"Good morning," the stranger says. She is younger, and her face is cheerful and friendly, her cheeks red from the cold outside.

"I'm looking for an address. I was told it was the third house on the left. I have a package for Darla."

This name rings no bells for you. But the woman looks chilled, and you want to help.

"Hmmm. I don't know who she is or where she lives, but it's definitely not for me. Come on in. I'll make a few phone calls; maybe we can figure this out together."

The woman comes in, and you put on a cup of tea. You begin to chat, and you quickly find you have more in common than you think. Though the topic of conversation itself is not particularly meaningful or deep, you find yourself invigorated by it.

You catch your reflection again in the mirror as you talk and feel somewhat embarrassed. You don't let on, hoping she doesn't notice the stark lack of effort put into your look today. You allow yourself to forget it, focusing instead on an unexpected friendship with a stranger.

After she leaves, you marvel at yourself for the first time in a very long time. What in the world had prompted you to invite this stranger into your home? You can't remember the last time you spent so long talking with someone you didn't know.

YOU FEEL ALIVE!

A world is waiting for you to explore it. There is more to life than the one you are living, and in all likelihood most of it won't come knocking at your door. With that said, it is that accessible—it just starts with you. Only you can make the decision to change your life.

When my husband was sick, really sick for an extended period of time, I too began showing symptoms of lifelessness, exhaustion, and illness. I gained weight. I wasn't sleeping. I wasn't eating well. I wasn't happy, and everything around me was suffering.

For some background, my husband, the man who swept me off my feet years ago worked in law enforcement for thirty-five years. He was an RCMP (Royal Canadian Mounted Police) officer and served his country well. There's more to that story, and you can read all about it in my book *My Life with a Cop: How to Survive the Ride.* We made it through an entire policing career together in one piece—a rare accomplishment!

We were so looking forward to travelling the world together in retirement. But as we were about to enter what should have been the best phase of our life, tragedy struck.

My husband, protector, provider, a man dedicated to taking care of his family, my lover and best friend, fell victim to post-traumatic stress disorder (PTSD). It was the darkest time in our lives. He became debilitated, dysfunctional, and depressed to the point of nearly committing suicide.

It was absolutely devastating. I became his caregiver, not his lover; his support system, not his friend; and his security, his rock. It was a long, lonely journey that was anything but easy. I'm happy to let you know it didn't last forever. He's doing really well, and with the culmination of heart, soul, mind, body, and strength we are loving life together again.

While I was immersed in taking care of my husband, I stopped taking care of myself. I was lonely. I was in a dark cloud that nearly consumed me. I began eating my emotions and turned to junk food for comfort. I stopped exercising, felt sluggish, and gained weight. I was miserable, unhealthy, and exhausted. Burned out!

One morning I woke up, and I knew I'd had enough. I didn't want to live like this anymore, and I was ready to make a change. From that moment onward, I was never the same.

Make this your moment, your "day one" on a journey to health, happiness, and absolute bliss. No matter where you are or what your life looks like, these steps can and will work for you. Are you ready to let your life begin again?

Investing in Yourself

Begin with this question: What are you doing to take care of yourself?

Honestly, I'd lived most of my life without even thinking of taking care of myself. When I asked myself this question for the first time, I flung my arms around my body and hugged myself to see if I would feel any different. I don't think anything happened, but I started to laugh. It hit me then that I hadn't laughed in a long time. I missed laughter in my life.

I decided at that moment that I was going to invest in myself. It's like when you're on an airplane and the flight attendants tell you to put on your own oxygen mask before you can help the person beside you. You're no good to anyone else if you can't breathe. In other words, you can't pour out of an empty cup. How could I go on taking care of my husband if I couldn't take care of myself?

And so my new life began. Similar to my wedding day, things have never been the same.

I ran to the washroom, turned on one of my favorite songs and blasted it. I climbed into the shower and started dancing under the spray, something I hadn't done in years. I sang along, letting myself smile and laugh and have fun. I felt as if I were washing away the old me, the me I didn't recognize, and getting ready to be the new, beautiful, and blissful me.

I blow-dried my hair, put on makeup, and threw on an outfit I looked good in, dressing up like I was going out to meet someone special. Hey, maybe I would! I was going to see the world through new eyes. I actually felt a little bit nervous.

I got in my car and glanced in the mirror. This time I didn't feel shame or embarrassment about my appearance. I was excited. My cheeks had color in them, my eyes were bright, and I was energized.

What does "self-care" or investing in yourself look like to you? Do you have fun? Do you take time for yourself, doing things you enjoy?

You can find so many ways to invest in yourself— whether it's going for a hike alone out in nature, taking yourself out for coffee, or buying a new pair of earrings. One of the most beneficial ways to invest in yourself is to find something that grows you, like watching personal development YouTube videos, reading books, or listening to podcasts.

Try a new hobby or interest, try a new recipe, and let yourself grow. Only you know what you and your body need. It's time to blast your favorite song, throw on your favorite outfit, and head out to explore the world.

I have a friend, Stephanie, who similarly made a dramatic change in her life. She was stuck in a rut and knew she needed to step out of her comfort zone and start living differently. For her first step she decided to challenge herself to talk to a stranger. Out running errands, she started to doubt herself but was determined not to return home until she had pushed herself.

Truth be told, she was terrified. She walked into a coffee shop full of people she didn't know and wondered what in the world she was thinking. How was she going to talk to a stranger? What would she even say? It would be so much easier to turn around and walk back outside.

This was Stephanie's first test. She knew if she didn't step out, she would give up completely. So she jumped. She proved to herself that she was committed to this. No turning back. Stephanie was ready to take a chance on change.

It was exhilarating. More than the conversation itself, the decision to be bold and follow through on the challenge Stephanie had given herself was thrilling. While that was only day one, Stephanie is now living a happy, healthy life.

You don't have to talk to a stranger as Stephanie did. But if you're serious about this, about really living, you will need to step out of your comfort zone. Prove to yourself that you're serious about this. Take the first steppingstone, right now, and let your life start all over again.

Believe it or not, people who invest in themselves are more successful. When I began this journey, I studied people who had what I was searching for, people who were loving life. I realized the main difference between their mindset and mine was that they spent time building into themselves.

Between reading books on personal growth, listening to wise and important, motivating voices, finding mentors in their lives, and hiring life coaches, they prioritized taking responsibility for their lives and their happiness.

It's your turn now. Stop settling for less than you deserve and make the decision to change your life. The best news here is that you're not alone in this. I'm going to give you my best secrets—recipes for joy, if you will, ladder rungs to climb for living your best life. All you have to do is jump.

Identifying Your Issues

Every spring, when the ground has thawed and the sun warms the air again, I make a habit of planting flowers around my deck. Digging deep in the ground, pushing past dirt, worms, and rocks to bury the seeds.

At first, it doesn't look like much. Then the rain falls, and they start to grow. Before long, I drink my morning coffee sitting on the deck, and when I do I can see them. The seeds in the dirt have grown, flourished, and become beautiful.

Truth be told, the journey of planting and growing flowers is not that different from the one we are beginning here.

Living a blissful life, starting over, and becoming the person you want to be will require you to take a good, hard look inward. You can't invest in yourself if you don't know who you are and what you need to work on.

There is not a person in the world who doesn't have room to grow—and the good news is, the more you start to take care of yourself, the easier it becomes. So first we're going to focus on digging deep to identify our own issues.

Let's Talk about Your Comfort Zone

Your comfort zone is exactly what it sounds like. Areas, relationships, and activities in your life that feel comfortable and safe. You don't have to push yourself to participate. It's where you retreat to if you're under stress or scared.

While feeling safe is important, simply put, you cannot grow if you are not challenged. If you won't push yourself, nothing will change. Auren Hoffman, an established and accomplished entrepreneur who has built five successful businesses, said the only way to maximize your learning is to spend seventy percent of your time doing hard things. While that sounds intimidating now, it's definitely motivating to get started.

For Stephanie, stepping out of her comfort zone was terrifying. Her heart was pounding, and she wanted to give up. But the rush and confidence she gained from her bold choice to talk to a stranger helped propel her forward. She's done much more stepping out since that first occasion, and as she's grown, her comfort zone has expanded with her.

When was the last time you stepped out of your comfort zone? Was it forced—or are you willing to choose to push yourself? Why do you think it's hard for you to step out of your comfort zone?

The fear of failure is one that is debilitating for many. Terrified of tripping and falling on their face, they give up before they even try. If there's one thing I've learned from all this, it's that falling forward is a good thing—and failure isn't always what it seems.

By this point in your life, you probably know that not everything goes according to plan. You've probably seen dominoes in action before—falling forward. Setting off a chain reaction of events. While dominoes are predictable by their predetermined route, life can be more unpredictable.

Isn't that what makes it wonderful? There are so many opportunities you haven't heard of yet, places you'll go where you never thought you could, and people you'll meet you didn't even know existed.

Find one way today in which you can push yourself to do something that scares you a little. Whether it's talking to a stranger, going out for coffee alone, calling up someone you haven't spoken to in years, or booking a trip to someplace you've never been.

Falling forward is still moving forward. Whether you're running, walking, or crawling along the ground toward what's ahead, the key is that you just keep moving. Be honest with yourself today. Are you willing to step out of your comfort zone? Are you ready to make a move for the good of your own future?

Let's Talk about Your Self-Confidence

When you walk into a room, how do you feel? Is your head held high? Are you focused on a person or a conversation? Do you walk in wondering what everyone thinks of you? Feeling self-conscious, overwhelmingly aware of people's facial expressions and body language toward you?

Can we be honest for a second? At this point in our lives, we've spent way too much time caring about the opinions of others. Once you hit sixty, it's long since time to let go of caring about what anyone else thinks of you.

Self-confidence is a lifelong battle for many women, but it doesn't have to be for you. You are a woman created and designed for greatness. It's time to start living as such. I can't promise everyone will like you, but I can tell you it doesn't matter. You were made for more. Let yourself off the hook—who cares what they think? Living for the approval of others will never get you where you want to be. This is your moment.

Every year, on New Year's Eve, countless women all over the world post/text/declare: "This is my year." I used to wonder what they meant by that. How would you know what a year would hold? Whether it would bring joy or pain, celebration or suffering? I understand now. This year, this month, this day can easily be yours if only you choose to reach out and take it. To stop living in the shadows.

Breaking long-standing habits of low self-confidence can be difficult, but there's never been a better time to start. Why not go out today? Find a power suit, new pair of jeans, fancy dress or new pair of heels—something you feel powerful in! Get yourself an extra confidence booster to throw on when you need it.

You own yourself, and you have unique talents and gifts the world needs to know about. You are a unique, creative individual, likely more so than you know yet. You were fearfully and wonderfully made to be exactly who you are and no one else.

Make this your year!

Let's Talk about Your Body Image

A 2013 study from the *Journal of Women and Aging* revealed that only 12 percent of women over fifty feel satisfied with their bodies.[2]

Are you in that 12 percent? When you look in the mirror, do you feel good about what you see?

Our culture has believed two huge lies. The first: beauty is defined by a size, scale number, or someone's opinion. The second: your worth is defined by beauty. We know we have a body image problem in our world, but we've tried to fix it using the wrong method. Telling someone they're beautiful doesn't fix their relationship with their body.

You see, your body wasn't designed only to be beautiful. It was designed to carry you through life. To hold you up, keep you moving. For many of us, it formed and gave us children. Your body has been with you every moment of your life. It can do incredible things, and it is not something we should be so hard on.

Body image is a sore spot for many of us, and an essential part of healing it is to trace back to the roots. While our culture may have believed lies about the body on the whole, most of us have accepted limiting beliefs about our individual bodies as well.

Denise grew up in a small town. She was surrounded by a loving family and close friends and was successful in nearly everything she did. She loved to skate, play hockey, and ride horses. She was, by all accounts, a tomboy and spent hours roaming the countryside with her friends.

Her body did incredible things. She had no reason to struggle with body image. As we all know, however, kids can be cruel. In elementary school, as a young child, an unkind classmate teased Denise, calling her "fat."

That one incident became an internalized belief that led to a severely unhealthy body image. For years, Denise hated looking in the mirror. She was anything but overweight, but the shame and humiliation she had felt didn't disappear. It wasn't until she was through her teenage years and well into adulthood that Denise began to realize she was so much more than her body. She began to love the skin she was in for the first time in a very long time.

If this has been a longstanding issue for you, it's worth asking the question of why. Have you been burned or lied to about your body? Has someone spoken something over you, declaring you are anything less than absolutely beautiful?

Don't let yourself be trapped by anyone else's standards anymore. Your body is part of you; it is everything you need it to be, and it was made specifically for you. You need it, and it needs you.

Let's Talk about Your Weight

Do you feel as if you could improve your health if you dropped a few pounds? Do you think it would make you happier? More satisfied?

The CDC reports that 49 percent of Americans try to lose weight at some point every year. We're immersed in weight-loss propaganda, between dieting products pitched left, right, and center; different fads and miracle foods claiming to work; and, of course, media that push us to assume a size zero is not only ideal, but average.

Maybe you're like Sara. Sara was one of those girls who grew up beautiful. She turned heads on the street, and when she walked into a room all eyes were on her. She was drop-dead gorgeous. As a teenager, she was told she should think about modelling. She was told she was certainly pretty enough, but she was just too heavy. Those words haunted Sara her entire life. Her weight became a never-ending struggle, a battle with herself to look like someone and something else.

The truth is that many of us could benefit our health by losing some weight. That's worth paying attention to, and it is certainly part of taking care of yourself; but it has to be done delicately. Do you want to lose weight for your health? To feel better, enjoy life more, and have more energy?

In order to take care of your body in a healthy way, you need to forgive yourself and others for the ways your body has been hurt. Sara needed to forgive herself and the person who had hurt her. By the grace of God, she learned she was beautiful; she was made in the image of God, as the Bible says; and she only needed to look like herself, like the beautiful woman God created.

Loving herself was the first step to a healthy weight-loss journey. It's time to stop believing the lies. You deserve a healthy, happy life. Believe it.

Releasing the hurts and letting go of the past are for your benefit. That will allow you to move forward in your life and hold your head high. When you can truly say you are thankful for who you are, you can move on to release the weight you want to lose through a healthy eating plan and love yourself the whole way through.

How Much Weight Do You Want to Lose?

When you are ready to take care of yourself physically and mentally, it's time to set some goals. If weight loss is one of them, coming up with a specific plan is a good guide both to help you and protect you from getting too sucked into the process.

I'm not a huge fan of the scale, particularly on weighing daily, but having starting numbers is important. It's worth recording where you are right now in order to celebrate your progress when you get there. If you're comfortable, you can even take "progress pictures" along the way, just for yourself, so you can visibly see the results instead of just the numbers.

Once you know where you're starting, it's time to set a goal weight. Be realistic and measurable with this. What is a healthy weight for your body type, height, and lifestyle? These are the questions you need to ask yourself honestly as you begin this journey, without getting overwhelmed.

Remember—this is about taking care of yourself, not about getting anyone else's approval. While you should keep realistic expectations about timing, remember healthy food choices and exercise will help you feel better almost overnight, even if they take a few weeks to be visible. You don't have to feel this way forever. You have an exciting and healthy, balanced future just ahead of you.

Keep in mind: The average American woman is a size twelve. Not a size zero. So take heart. Your first goal on your weight-loss journey is simply to start eating healthier and feeling better about what you are putting into your body. Add regular exercise into your routine, like going for a walk once or twice a day. This shouldn't be something that feels intimidating. You are giving your body the attention it deserves. It's carrying a powerful woman, and it's time to make sure she's properly equipped.

What Are Your Relationship Goals?

People were made for each other. Whether married or single, living in a busy city or the quiet countryside, every single one of us needs and craves some kind of community. It's in our wiring.

The experience of losing one of my best friends has led me to look at friendships through a different lens. True kindred spirits are hard to find, and the loss of a friendship is one that must be grieved deeply. Despite this, it's allowed me to examine other relationships in my life, my own behavior in friendships, and how to build strong ones moving forward.

Take out a sheet of paper and make a list of how many good friends you have. Not just acquaintances or casual friends, but people who really know you and you know you can rely on. What do you want to build, either in those relationships or in new ones entirely? Are you hoping for deeper relationships or just more of them? Looking to meet like-minded people or friends to have over for dinner?

Before you can create the kind of relationships you want, you need a vision for them. Once you have an idea, it's time to create an action plan of how to achieve them.

If you're looking to meet like-minded people, try finding groups to join, events to attend, or places to go where you're likely to make those kinds of connections. If you're hoping to have friends you can have over for dinner, call them and invite them over for dinner! Reach out to people you haven't talked to in a while.

Meeting people usually means stepping out of your comfort zone and making yourself a little uncomfortable. Authentic relationships require vulnerability and sacrifice. If you want friends who are there for you, you need to be there for them first. Think of the Golden Rule in this scenario: *"Do unto Others as You Would Have Others Do unto You."*[3]

You will have to push yourself, but it will be so rewarding. A fool-proof trick you can try is to walk up to someone in a coffee shop, grocery store, or church and find a way to compliment them. "I love those shoes!" "Where did you get that top?" "Cute earrings!" "Love your hair!" Women love to hear things like that, and it's a great ice breaker and way to open up a conversation without requiring a long one if they seem busy or uninterested.

Loneliness is an incredibly painful thing to walk through. For those of you who are married, you're probably well aware that saying "I do" doesn't save you from feeling alone, even within your marriage. Spending your life with someone is an incredibly beautiful thing to do, but finding yourself in seasons of distance is common.

What do you want out of your marriage? Where is it now? On the other side of that same piece of paper, make a list of positive characteristics in marriage. Examples may include: good communication, healthy sex life, having fun together, and friendship. Yes, friendship. The foundation to any happy marriage or relationship. If you are not friends with your spouse, if you don't enjoy their company or person, it's time to have a serious look at making some changes in your relationship. By no means am I suggesting you give up! Only that it might be worth adding some new practices and habits into your relationship.

In all likelihood, if you're miserable, your marriage is probably struggling. If either partner feels dissatisfied, it's almost certain that would affect the other. Reigniting excitement in your relationships is probably easier than you think and can be as simple as planning a fun date night for the first time in a while. Get dressed in something that makes you feel desirable and go have fun with your partner. You never know what will happen later!

Discover things you like doing together and make an effort to do them regularly. Ask each other new questions. Go on a trip together, even just a weekend getaway. You can even work on making friends together and building a community to support not just you individually, but your marriage.

With these goals in mind and action steps to take, make the commitment right now to invest in yourself. In your passions, in your growth, and in your relationships. Launch yourself confidently into this new phase of your life. You're beginning a thrilling stage, a new adventure in your sixties. Don't you dare turn back now!

Chapter 2

Making a Plan

Years ago, I signed up as a member at a women's gym. I fell in love with it almost instantly. The workouts, community, encouragement, and simplicity of it were amazing. I knew right away I didn't just want to be a part of it; I wanted to have my own Curves gym.

I began to dream. I thought about it, talked about it, and created a vision. This was a huge goal, and if I wanted to see it realized I needed an actual plan. The gym I attended was a territory franchise, meaning I couldn't open another one in my city. I refused to give up and began to look into opening a location in my hometown, which was seven hours away from where I lived at the time. I began the process and soon was faced with the choice to go all-in and commit to the process or give up on my goal altogether.

I'm thankful I committed, and I've never looked back. It took six months of blood, sweat, and tears from my husband and me, a lot of hard work and dedication—

but we did it. That one decision changed my life. This experience was what taught me about nutrition, exercise, and motivating women just like you. I loved my work, the women I got to know, and being able to support them on every step of their journeys. I got to see them transform their entire lives, getting the results they were looking for, finding the relationships they craved, loving themselves for the first time and having the faith they deeply desired.

All of those women believed in themselves again. They believed their lives could begin again.

Fitness Goals

Now that you're in, committed, and ready to change your life, it's time to get moving. In order to do this effectively and create lasting habits, we need to start with a plan.

Take some time to think about what your end result is. Do you want to be able to walk five km comfortably? Do you want to run a marathon? Do you want to be able to play with your grandkids on the floor? Do you want to complete twenty pushups?

Once you have a vision for the results you want, it's time to set your goals! Each goal is a small step you will take toward achieving your end result. This means it's important to set the right goals. If you've never done a pushup before, don't challenge yourself to drop and do fifty today. I like to set what are called MTO goals. It's a technique my coach taught me, and implementing it has been extremely helpful.

"MTO" stands for minimum, target, outrageous. If you don't exercise regularly, your first goal might be to go to the store and outfit yourself for what you'll need for your fitness goals. This might be your minimum goal: purchasing a pair of runners. Then your target goal might be to go for a ten-minute walk once this week. If you've never done any exercise before, doing those two things is a great start!

Your outrageous goal might be to go for a brisk ten-minute walk five times this week! You get the idea—give yourself realistic goals you can accomplish and celebrate. Challenge yourself with targets you can actually hit. This will help you stay motivated as you work toward what you want. Don't worry about where anyone else is; your goals are individual and unique to you.

So what kind of exercise sounds fun to you? Swimming, dancing, running, tennis? Does going to a gym sound exciting, or do you like the idea of working out at home? Do you enjoy going for walks and taking in nature scenery, or would you have more fun throwing on a movie and walking on a treadmill from your own home?

Exercise can (and should) be fun! You have so many different ways to move your body, from quiet strolls to tennis matches, or maybe it's all-out dancing in your living room. But it's worth finding something you enjoy doing and starting there. Remember, you're doing this to increase your happiness, so find something that does just that.

The MTO goal-setting process works for every aspect of your life. We're going to be following this system, so have fun with it. Let yourself dream and really plan where you want to be. Big vision means big payoff, and you need to know what you're working toward.

Nutrition and Weight-Loss Goals

Following the same principle, you need to define for yourself what your nutrition and weight-loss goals are. Do you want to maintain your weight, build muscle, gain or lose weight? Are you focused on healthy living for the feeling of having more energy or being able to fit into your jeans?

When I was in elementary school, my mother used to pack me "healthy" lunches. I'm sure they were very nutritious, but as a child I had no interest in lunches with no treats. One particular day I watched a friend of mine pull out some beautiful, rich, chocolate cake. I wanted that chocolate cake, and I wanted it badly. I spent a couple of moments working up the courage to ask if I could have a piece. He must've taken pity on me because, shockingly enough, he said yes!

The important point here is that the only way you're going to get what you want is if you ask for it. It takes courage to be honest about what you want out of life, but you are the only one who can make it happen.

Personal goals like weight loss and nutrition are most easily reached when you are surrounded by support. Accountability is a huge component of any goal, and finding either an individual or a group of people who can hold you to your plan will make a world of difference.

You don't want someone who will make you feel bad or dejected about making a mistake; you will slip up occasionally, and that's okay. But you need someone who can motivate you and keep you on track and whose opinion you value. You will need some tough love at times! It's easy enough to tell a stranger what your goals are, but you need to pick someone you trust and feel safe with so you can celebrate your successes and allow them to kick you in the butt when necessary as you go through your journey.

Set up an actual connection plan: whether it's weighing in and calling your accountability partner once a week to tell them your results, letting them know every time you head to exercise, or sending them your meal plan for the week to keep up your healthy nutrition. Make sure you give yourself concrete and doable action steps.

Tip: Write down all the goals and steps you set for yourself. It will make you feel better to cross them off as you go and help you see your progress and your end result!

Eating healthy is commonly mislabeled as missing out on good food. The truth is that a healthy lifestyle is all about balance, and you can find fun ways to eat foods that won't hurt your body and you won't be missing out.

Here's a quick tip: Throw some grapes in the freezer. When you're craving something sweet, grab a few—they taste like candy, only with a lot less sugar and none of the processed chemicals.

For me, living a happy, healthy life means I want to make the most of every second. We never know what the future holds, and I don't want to waste my time. Yesterday is gone, and tomorrow isn't guaranteed—let's strive to make each day count.

You're getting back on track here. Before long, your target goals will feel more like your minimum goals—and maybe you'll even be hitting your outrageous goals.

I have a good friend, Joan. She's one of those wonderfully upbeat people. But when I met her she was feeling pretty blah about herself. She was self-conscious, lacking confidence, and desperate to achieve and maintain her ideal weight. Joan knew what she wanted, but she didn't know how to get there.

The two of us sat down and created an entire blueprint. We worked hard to come up with a plan to achieve exactly what she wanted, and she began sprinting toward it. She never took her eyes off her target and hit it dead center. Not only did Joan lose a hundred pounds, but her life was completely changed. She was happy with herself and her life for the first time in a long time.

This is your future. It may seem like a long road ahead, but it's only a short jump to the next step, and the ending is so worth it.

Challenge: Start journaling your eating habits! Write down what you can remember eating for the last two weeks and keep a record of everything you eat for the next two weeks. Not only will this help you be aware of what you're putting into your body; but it will also keep you accountable, and you can see the change in what you're eating as you become more focused on health. Be honest and admit to yourself what you put in your body, whether it is good, bad, or ugly!

Relationship Goals

In order to feel as if I'm fulfilled in my life, I need relationships. I don't need a huge circle, but having those two or three go-to friends I can call up at any time and hang out with when I need my woman-to-woman fix makes a difference.

Just like with fitness and nutrition, it's time to set some goals for your relationships. It takes planning and effort, like anything else, so get real and ask yourself what you want.

Often, relationship goals mean digging a little deeper with each step, becoming more vulnerable and addressing things you may not want to admit about yourself. It's not easy, but it will enrich your current relationships and make new ones so much stronger. This very book was developed by my digging through my own dirt, and I can confidently tell you it was so worth it!

What do you want out of a relationship? Do you want fun, support, encouragement? Do you want new adventure? Do you want to go out for lunch and have deep discussions over controversial topics? Different friends will meet different needs for all of us, so make sure you know what you're searching for.

Your goal might be to develop the relationship you have with your spouse. You can do this alongside developing other friendships, or maybe you want to focus on that goal right now.

As you begin those steps, you need to take note of the fact that you can only change yourself. You cannot control your spouse or a friend, for that matter. If you want to improve your relationship, you need to recognize you can improve only your own behavior—without expectation for your partner to follow suit. More often than not, when you change your responses and reactions, your spouse will do the same. You can't, however, expect them to read your mind or get everything right.

Challenge: Make this a game for yourself. Pick things you can do each day for your spouse: a surprise, a compliment, something that will make him smile or totally shock him. Have fun with it and enjoy taking time to serve your spouse and your relationship. Watch it play out and see what happens!

Boundaries in Relationships

When you're in a close relationship with someone, it's easy to adopt their habits, both positive and negative. While you are on this journey of personal development, it is essential to set boundaries in both friendships and spousal relationships to ensure that your growth is not sabotaged. Sometimes, people who love you the most give the worst advice and can be negative sources as you challenge yourself.

For example, your weight-loss plan or nutrition plan may not line up with how your spouse wants to eat or live. It's important to be comfortable saying no and, if you need to, doing something for yourself even if people don't understand it.

Relationships and friendships don't mean always seeing eye-to-eye. People will disagree, and that's okay. Being able to share conflicting perspectives with mutual respect and agree to disagree is actually a really important part of a strong friendship. Friendships, at the core, are developed by strangers sharing perspectives and opinions with each other at increasing degrees of intimacy. When is the last time you met a new friend and actually developed that relationship? It takes time to get to know someone on a deep level.

Ask yourself this: If you could improve one thing in an important relationship you have now, what would that be?

I asked my friend Rhonda this recently. Without hesitation she told me she needed to let go of a close friendship or at the very least set some boundaries because she was heading down a dangerous path. A close friend of hers was going through a difficult time and coping with it by regularly going out drinking. She would phone Rhonda late at night on her way to the bar, begging Rhonda to join her for support. Tired and miserable, Rhonda knew this was not a healthy pattern.

As she began to think about it, Rhonda realized she needed to set a boundary for herself and tell her friend she could no longer continue to support her in this way. She would always love and support her, but not by encouraging her to drink her problems away. Not only was this making it worse, Rhonda was being dragged down with her.

You've probably heard it said that you are an average of the five people with whom you spend the most time. Who are those five people in your life? Write down their names and get real with yourself. Write down the characteristics you respect about them and the ones you feel are hurting you. Are they people you admire and want to be like, or do you need to take a step back from certain relationships?

It's time to set your relationship goals. Minimum, target, and outrageous—plan out your steps and get going. Have fun digging!

Chapter 3

Changing Your Mindset

Negative Outlook vs Positive Outlook

For as he thinks in his heart, so is he (Proverbs 23:7).[4]

It is no secret that the way you look at your life has a drastic impact on the outcome of your life. With this in mind, if you really want to change your life, you will have to change your mindset.

Focusing on the negative around you will get you negative results. A positive outlook, however—choosing to see the good around you and believing the best about yourself—will lead to happiness and the life you want.

On average, we have between fifty thousand to eighty thousand thoughts every day. If the bulk of those are negative, that's a huge weight to bear. Research shows that on average the ratio of negative to positive thoughts for an individual is between nine to one and five to one.

This is astounding. That's a lot of negativity, and it takes a lot of positive thinking and intentionality to alter your thought patterns, but it needs to happen. Your thoughts don't just stay thoughts. They become things, which lead to action, and action leads to results. If you are constantly overwhelmed by negative thoughts, those negative thoughts will bring you negative results. Whatever goes through your mind will expand and become your reality in one way or another, so be careful with what you choose to let in.

Having a confident mindset also allows you to hear other perspectives in healthy ways. Talking to people with different worldviews, values, and lifestyles allows you to grow in really important ways. It enables you to see things you couldn't see before and can spark inspiration and imagination.

Positivity can be misconstrued as unrealistic and overly optimistic, but having a healthy outlook on life doesn't mean pretending bad things don't exist. It's just choosing not to focus on them. It's letting go of the things you can't control and approaching the ones you can with action and determination rather than fear. Optimistic people live longer too!

Negativity leads to self-doubt. Doubt is the devil's most prized possession—because if you are immersed in it you're frozen, at a standstill. You can't possibly move forward if you're second-guessing every move you make. Doubt paralyzes you and keeps you from becoming the woman you were meant to be. It's time to shut down the nasty voice in your head and step into a happy, healthy life.

This is a crucial piece to the puzzle. Please do not miss this step. Even if you changed your circumstances entirely, without a mind shift, you likely won't be any happier. Changing the way you see things can alter the entire trajectory of your life very quickly, so waste no time.

Self-Love

What is self-love?

Self-love is a pretty hot topic right now, and it seems like everyone's got their own definition or interpretation of what it means. I believe two popular conceptualizations of self-love are important to address.

First, that self-love is self-centered, egotistical, and vain. A disregard for those around you. I strongly disagree with this view.

The other is that self-love is a necessity and something you do to take care of yourself. I strongly do agree with this view. In order to become the woman you want to be, you need to take care of yourself. If you aren't caring for and protecting yourself and your needs, not only will you be miserable, but you can't do anything for anyone around you. Your suffering will only hurt your spouse, children, and friends, and you will burn out. Maybe you already have. If you feel selfish or guilty for trying to take care of yourself, you need to dismiss those feelings right now. Put them behind you and don't look back! Not only is it okay to practice self-love; it is healthy and necessary to live a full life.

Don't change your life because you don't like yourself. Do it because you love yourself. Don't try to shed the pounds because you hate your body—do it because you love it.

When my husband fell ill with PTSD (post-traumatic stress disorder) I stopped taking care of myself. Between his mental illness and my own exhaustion, things were getting worse and worse. I was at the end of my rope when I finally realized that if I didn't take care of myself I could do nothing for him.

His mental illness was the greatest barrier either of us had ever gone through, and as awful as it was, the experience ended up being one of my greatest strengths. Not only am I able to help others going through something similar now, but it was also in that season I learned how to love myself.

Starting to practice self-care after a long time away can be hard. At first, people questioned my actions, and it was painful. I was looked down on and criticized for trying to take care of myself. While that initially made me doubt myself, I fought to trust my intuition, and I came out stronger because of it. Things changed, and the very people who had critiqued my choices realized the difference wasn't just in my life. Taking care of myself meant we were both doing better, and it was a huge step on the road to recovery.

At one point in the middle of it I had to make a choice to put the negative thoughts behind me. I had to set strong boundaries in relationships and refuse to listen to the naysayers. I had to buckle down, focus on my determination, and continue on my plan until every goal was met.

Changing my mindset about loving myself was an important shift. You may not love where you are right now, and that's okay. But in order to live a happy and healthy life you need to choose to love who you are right now so you can love your life later.

Shake off the guilt and any voices that say self-care is selfish—they're lying to you. It's time to start saying yes to yourself, believing your future is bright and knowing God wants more for you.

Gratitude

Maybe one of the most important steps you'll take in changing your mindset is gratitude. If you don't already have a gratitude journal, you need to start one. This is not something you should put off. Grab a piece of paper and a pen and start by writing one sentence about something you are grateful for.

Try to think outside of easy grade-school answers. What about your body? Even if you don't love it right now, it does so many wonderful things, without which life would be so different. I'm sure you are grateful your lungs expand and allow you to breathe.

Here are a few examples to get you started.

I am grateful for my legs that move and allow me to walk.

I am grateful for my eyes that allow me to see the beautiful colors all around me.

I am grateful for my ears that let me hear the birds sing.

I am grateful for my nose so I can smell the delicious aromas of food I prepare.

I am grateful for my tastebuds that allow me to enjoy the healthy food I prepare.

I am grateful for my warm bed to sleep in at night.

I am grateful for my pillow to lay my head on.

I am grateful for my safe home to live in.

I am grateful for clean water to drink.

I am grateful for my family, my children and grandchildren.

You can always find something for which to be grateful. The more you practice gratitude, the easier it becomes. Stop and write down something you are grateful for right now—even before you read any further.

Believe it or not, gratitude is an essential part of happiness. It's been so life-changing for me that it's become part of my morning routine. I start off every single day writing in my gratitude journal. It may take you a few weeks to get into the habit, but I can promise you that starting off your day being thankful for what you have will reframe your entire day.

Gratitude fuels my creativity. It helps me think outside the box, coming up with more and more things for which to be grateful.

A few years ago I met a young woman named Janet. She was a student from China who came to study at the university in my city. We met while she was here, and she decided I should be her "Mom." Janet was young and enthusiastic, and no one loved life as she did.

She loved learning and was grateful for every opportunity to do so. She was always excited to come over, to see how I cooked, to learn English better, and to eat with my family. She was eager to cook and share her recipes also, and she loved spending time with me.

Janet's zest for life resulted from her grateful nature. She was thankful for every good thing and every fun evening, and she was so delightful to be around. Everyone loved having Janet in their presence, and her positive spirit was a huge component to her success as she became a powerful businesswoman. Her grateful heart was one that not only made her happier, but helped propel her closer to her career goals.

Being grateful for the things around you can change your entire world, just as it did for Janet. It can bring you opportunities and relationships, and even if it doesn't, you'll be much happier right where you are.

Did you know that when you look up to the ceiling you can't frown? Not only is this a great pick-me-up tool, but it's also a great life lesson. If you keep your eyes focused upward, on the good things ahead of you, the new heights you're going to reach, you won't be miserable. It's only when you start to look down, on yourself or others, that things fall apart.

Growth Mindset

A huge asset on this journey will be developing a "growth mindset." You need to determine how you see yourself. If you are stuck in your old ways and see no value in looking at different perspectives, it's kind of like living in a closed box. You have no light and no oxygen, and inevitably you live out a slow and painful death.

The good news is that the box has a lid, and it's one you can take off. When you open the box, the walls part. There is no limit, and you can breathe, grow, and become more than you knew was possible.

People who have a growth mindset will never stop improving themselves. They want to be the best version of themselves. They see learning as a way to success and see obstacles as a way to keep learning. They embrace challenges, are determined to find solutions rather than giving up or quitting, and go after what they want.

To grow, you have to give yourself room. An oak tree doesn't fit in a window planter. You have to believe you can go where you want to go and create space for the person you are becoming.

Be willing to learn, grow, and be challenged. Try new things! Whether it's new recipes, foods, exercises, friends, or cities—step out of your routine a little and see what else is out there.

You have talents and gifts that can and should be expanded on. Don't let a fixed mindset shrink you or hold you back. Have you heard it said that your greatest barrier is ultimately your greatest success? It's true—the bigger the challenge, the bigger the reward. Right now, I encourage you to open your mind to a new world. Don't just think outside the box; live outside it too. You have no idea what you're capable of yet, and it's time for us all to find out. The world is ready for you.

Self-Talk

We've all heard the saying "sticks and stones may break my bones, but words will never hurt me." That statement is a lie. In fact, the words we hear about ourselves play a huge role in who we become and the things we repeat.

When I was in elementary school, one of my peers told me I was fat. This was at a time when I was beginning to notice boys, develop crushes, and spend days trying to get them to notice me too. Those words stuck with me for years. I played them over and over in my mind. In adulthood I thought I had dealt with the issue. But when I gained weight with my first pregnancy those harsh words and the self-criticism came rushing back.

The way you talk to yourself is extremely important. Nearly all of the time, we are harder on ourselves than we would ever be on anyone else. We have ridiculous ideas about beauty, worth, and the way people see us that likely have very little bearing on the truth.

It takes a lot of work to change long-standing thought patterns, but this is one of the most important things you'll ever do. Learning to cut yourself some slack, be content with who you were made to be, and appreciate your individual identity will change your life like nothing else.

Whether you're critiquing your own physical appearance, personality, talents, or lack thereof, it needs to stop today. You weren't meant to be anyone else—only you. And you deserve to live the happiest, healthiest, fullest version of your life you possibly can.

Let's Talk about Stress

Stress plays a huge role in your mindset. Let's take a look at what it means and how you can deal with it in healthy ways.

Defining the Problem.

There are two types of stress: eustress and distress. To keep things simple, I'm going to call them "good stress" and "bad stress." Bad stress can be split further into two categories: acute and chronic.

Stress is actually your body's natural response to help you overcome challenges in your life, not to create them. When you are able to channel that stress into an appropriate response, it allows your body to make a wise decision and act accordingly.

It could look something like this: You are stressed because you have to make a quick business decision, and it carries a lot of weight. You list the pros and cons, and they are pretty much balanced, so you have to go with your own intuition. You know in your gut what feels right, so you make the call. You don't hesitate because you know hesitation hurts. Before you know it your work has paid off, and you have doubled your income! This is good stress.

When you are unable to channel that stress into an appropriate response, however, it quickly causes problems in your life, and soon your body suffers. You are not handling your stress. You can't let it go. You go to bed, and your mind does not let you forget that conflict you had at work. Your mind is reeling, and you keep worrying about what the rest of your staff will think of you. You doubt your decision, a headache sets in, and you're up all night. This snowballs into a pattern until your mental and physical health is in jeopardy. Stress is a huge factor in health issues and weight gain. It sends your body into panic mode and prevents you from being able to achieve the healthy lifestyle you so desire.

Coping.

How do you cope with stress? Do you manage it, or does it manage you? A huge cause of stress for many people is the unconscious habit of comparing themselves with the people around them.

There's that person—someone who always has it together. They're detail oriented, outgoing, and active and make things happen. Who wouldn't wish to be like them?

The danger of comparison is that you never know what's really going on. The person you are comparing yourself to could be on the edge of a breakdown, people pleasing to the point of self-destruction. They may not be able to rest or set boundaries, be terrified of failure, and lack balance in their lives.

If this describes you, if you feel like you're burning the candle at both ends, you are putting yourself at risk, and the results can be devastating. My husband's PTSD was caused by years of stress that wasn't dealt with, and while he has made almost a full recovery, not everyone does. It can be completely debilitating, and I cannot stress enough the importance of finding balance in your life.

Meditation.

Meditation is one of the most effective ways to relieve stress. It allows you to clear your mind, almost like a palate cleanser, opening it up to new levels of peace and creativity.

Practicing meditation is like a body detox or a cleanse. In the same way your body needs to be cleansed of toxins, so does your mind. Many poisons are flooding it. If you don't remove them, they halt your creativity, emotional stability, and clear thought process.

Next time you're overwhelmed or in need of a fresh start, try meditating before anything else. Let your mind be clear so you have nothing holding you back. You can start anew and allow your mind to tap into whatever it is you need to focus on from a more stable and solid place.

Tapping/Emotional Freedom Technique (EFT).
Tapping or EFT is an easy tool that involves using your fingers to tap on particular points on the body which allow it to release stress and painful emotions.

When you practice tapping, you focus on the present moment. Step one of this technique is to identify your stress level on a one-to-ten scale before you begin. As you tap these meridian points, it can significantly bring down that level. Every notch back to zero is another added bonus. If this interests you, you will find many great resources on YouTube about this technique, and I encourage you to research it for yourself (some self-love).

Visualization.
Visualization is not only a great tool for stress, but it's a great way to start the day before you even get out of bed.

The key to visualization is to self-fulfill whatever prophecies you set for yourself. If you expect and visualize feeling exhausted and frustrated, and everything seems to be falling apart, you'll likely experience that in reality. When you wake up in the morning, look at yourself right then, as you are cozy in bed, and visualize yourself all done up from head to toe—favorite outfit, looking dazzling and ready to meet whatever your day holds.

This doesn't need to take long, but it can help you go into your day feeling prepared and positive. If you have a stressful meeting or proposal for work, visualize walking into a positive and exciting outcome, rather than dreading it and walking in nervously.

Take the next conflict or stressful event you know you have coming up, and sit and visualize a positive outcome for at least five minutes before entering that circumstance. The point is to visualize positively and get your mind focused on the good and the potential of a good outcome versus focusing on the negative outcome. What you focus on expands.

Visualization can change your life. I met a lady from Colombia who read my book *Renew Your Mind: Maximize Your Potential*. As soon as she started following some of the guidelines I set out, she realized this would change her life and began immediately to implement visualization into her daily routine.

Every morning when she wakes up, she envisions her day and all of the good things it could hold. Her life has improved so much, and her entire perspective on it has shifted simply because she takes a few minutes every morning to reset her expectations.

Reading.

Reading is a fantastic exercise to calm your mind. When you get lost in a book, your brain can't wander off to stress and overthink.

Reading the Bible is something that often works for me. I love reading in the Psalms especially if I'm stressed. The prayers bring me so much comfort and peace and allow me to give my cares to God every day.

Matthew 6:25-27[5] says: "Therefore I tell you, do not worry about your life, what you will eat or drink; or about your body, what you will wear. Is not life more than food, and the body more than clothes? Look at the birds of the air; they do not sow or reap or store away in barns, and yet your heavenly Father feeds them. Are you not much more valuable than they? Can any one of you by worrying add a single hour to your life?"

When's the last time you read a good book you couldn't put down? It may be time to pick up another one. Also, countless books offer tips to help motivate you on this journey.

With each book you read, challenge yourself to remember a quote, a one-liner, a story, or a piece of information that stands out. Write it down if you need to. Words can entirely redefine your life and are things you can come back to and rely on when you need them.

I once heard someone describe reading Scripture as digging a well for yourself. Regardless of whether or not you feel like you're "getting something" out of each read, you're deepening the well. When life gets tough and complicated, you can draw from what you know and what you have stored up.

I love something a coach of mine told me, and I've kept it in my mind for a long time: "A drop of ink in a sea of milk is still a sea of milk."[6]

This is something I rely on and come back to in the face of failure or mistakes. A slip up or flaw is still just a drop in the sea that is your life and your legacy. It doesn't have to define it any more than any other drop would. Books and words contain so much wisdom and are an extremely beneficial tool for relaxation and refocusing in stressful times.

Listening to Podcasts.
For those of you who aren't big readers—or if you've got a long commute or drive coming up—you have a great opportunity to take advantage of the world of podcasts, videos, and online resources.

Zig Ziglar, a great motivational speaker I had the pleasure of meeting, used to say he did a lot of learning through "automobile university." If one person in the world had a zest for life, it was Zig. He always saw the cup as not just half full, but overflowing.

It's estimated that the average American spends more than eight hours a week in their car. You can spend that time in silence or listening to the radio, or you can choose to dedicate that time to bettering and educating yourself in automobile university.

Particularly in this day and age, countless podcasts, audiobooks, and YouTube videos are filled with motivation, personal development material, or new skills you can learn simply by driving home. It's a healthy challenge to try to learn something new every day, whether that's part of a new language, leadership skills, or new ideas for your fitness and relationship goals. You can find information dedicated to every topic in the world, and now that you've established the goals you want to hit in your life, you can find sources tailored to those needs.

Listening to different ideas and perspectives helps you have some "aha" moments. It broadens your horizons and allows you to open up your eyes and see things you couldn't before. You may not agree with everything you listen to, and that's okay. It's important to have your own voice. Hearing conflicting opinions may actually deepen and inform your own or even help you develop a passion for something you never knew you cared about.

My friend Jenny listens to Oprah every day while she commutes to work. She says the topic, whatever it is, makes her think. When she gets to work, she always has a different question to ask one of her colleagues. It engages her own mind and those of the people around her, gives her an automatic conversation starter, and adds some excitement to her life.

Check out a podcast and you'll have an automatic "in" with a stranger while you stand in a line or sit in a coffee shop. Maybe you'll be on the phone with a long-time friend you haven't talked to in a while or even sitting down to dinner with your spouse and don't want to run out of things to talk about. Learning new things will make it easier to spark a conversation, and you'll find yourself more frequently engaged in long, interesting discussions.

Being in Nature.

Getting outside, being in nature, and soaking up the world around you is an unparalleled boost for your body, brain, and soul. Nature grounds you and is key for your "mental fitness." Mental fitness means the ability to have a positive sense of how you think, feel, and act, which improves your ability to enjoy life! Being in nature gives you a reset, a reminder of how big the world is, and helps you to process your emotions.

Sandra, a friend of mine, recently went on a trip to Cancun. She went for a walk on the beach, one that stretched for miles and miles. She talked about how white the sand was and the way it felt between her toes. When she stopped, she could feel every little granule as her feet sank into the soft, smooth surface. As she stood there, Sandra realized the granules didn't help her stand straight. Her alignment was off.

This simple moment provided a huge wake-up call for her. When she stood still, became stagnant, her life wasn't aligned with where she wanted to be. She needed to keep moving and pushing herself. Growth is a journey that never ends. Truth is, if you're not actively learning and growing, you are dying.

While this is just one lesson that came out of the beauty of nature, being in it will always bring you back to yourself. Let yourself breathe fresh air, feel the sand between your toes, and enjoy the mountains. It is inarguably one of the greatest sources of bliss in my life.

There is a serenity that comes only with the stillness of the world. A quiet evening on the ocean, the wind whistling through the trees, even a cozy evening during a thunderstorm. The outdoor world serves as a reminder that no matter what pain or turmoil you've endured, you can always find beauty.

When you truly love yourself and find real contentment, it's pure pleasure that overflows your heart with gratitude.

Your heart and soul become one with nature, and you feel true love, joy, and peace.

Strategies for Stress

Many strategies can help you manage your stress, but here are a few I use that work well for me. Let's start with the Pattern Interrupt. This is where you select a specific word—such as shift, change, transition, move, interrupt. When you feel yourself getting overwhelmed or stressed out, you say this word out loud and consciously allow it to interrupt your thoughts. Say to yourself, "That was then; this is now."

Another strategy is to focus on the Present Moment. Right now hold something that grounds you, like a rock, a flower, even a twig from outside. Feel it, and use your senses to bring you into the present moment. Does this thing you are holding have a color? Does it smell? Does it make a noise or a sound when you tap it? How does it feel, and what is its texture? Can you taste it?

You could also use a lemon or an orange. This is my favorite way of getting into the present moment. Hold the lemon—look at its color. It makes me smile because yellow is a sign of brightness and light. Now feel the lemon. Run your fingers across its surface. It is smooth, a little bumpy, and kind of round. Next, break the skin or peel the lemon. What do you hear as you peel it? What do you smell now?

And then taste it—do you pucker up and make a face? Or is it sweet to your taste buds?

Go outside if you can and take off your socks to feel the ground beneath your feet. Think about your senses. How does the ground feel? Is it cold, warm, hot, smooth, rough, prickly, itchy, textured, pebbled, sandy, comfortable? What do you see? What do you smell? What do you feel? What do you taste? What do you hear?

Another thing to try is Tactical Breathing. This is a time-honored technique used in a war setting where there was no beautiful music, no peaceful ocean waves, no soothing aroma to soak in. No, there were only the sounds of gunshots, people screaming, orders barked; and yet this time-honored tool worked to help people focus on the present.

Breathe in deeply, and as you inhale count to four. As you do so, visualize the numbers; focus on them. Then hold your breath for the count of four and repeat visualizing the numbers. Now exhale fully to the count of four, again visualizing the numbers, and last hold for four counts visualizing the numbers. Repeat again from the beginning. With each count, try to see the numbers in your mind. Do this deep breathing exercise three to five times and practice this technique whenever you think about it. Soon you will be able to do this exercise anywhere, anytime and any place inconspicuously.

It's easy to feel as if there's no escape from stress. As if it will be with you forever, almost as if it's part of you. But you don't have to live that way. No matter what's going on around you, it's time to take control of your emotional well-being. Mental health is every bit as important as physical health, and neither one can be fully achieved without the other. No more living in fear or stress—you've got this.

Chapter 4

Physical Exercise

Starting to exercise in your sixties can sound almost ridiculous. It's hard work, right? You're sixty, maybe retired, and this is when you planned on taking it easy and just enjoying life, right?

Here's the thing: It's true what they say. You are as young as you feel. I'm sixty, but I feel forty. I'm not retired—I'm refired! I'm renewed and living a more fulfilling life than ever before. I'm sixty, and it's because I care about enjoying life that I exercise. I want to play with my grandkids, enjoy travelling, and be able to carry my suitcase up the stairs by myself.

I want to be flexible and be able to run up and down the stairs if I'm in a rush. I want to go on cruises, see the world, and be strong enough to make the most of it. I don't want to run out of steam before I can accomplish these things. And if I don't keep up with exercise, that's a very real possibility.

So whether or not I'm "in the mood" I will work out. It doesn't have to be a chore; soon enough, it becomes a habit and something you'll enjoy. When you feel and see the changes it makes in your life, you'll never want to give it up.

Gym or Home Workouts

The first step is to decide where you're going to work out. Luckily, you have many options and resources for both gym and home workouts. Each option has pros and cons; it just comes down to preference.

If you need to work out around other people to be motivated, sign up for a gym membership. If you feel uncomfortable working out with others and get enough community elsewhere, then try working out at home. Either way, you're going to feel better and stronger in no time.

Once you've figured that out, you'll want to pick up a couple of things. Get some good runners, a Yoga mat (if you're working out at home), and a cute gym outfit. Make sure you get something you feel good in! Have fun with it. When you have your outfit on, music going, and water in hand, you'll know you're ready to exercise.

Explore different workout styles! Do you like using weights or prefer calisthenics (using your own body weight)? Both are great options. I prefer using my own body weight—doing things like pushups, lunges, burpees, jumping jacks and, of course, the dreaded plank.

If neither of those sounds appealing, try something like swimming, walking, biking, dancing, running or whatever you think you'll enjoy and want to add to your life. Find something you can stick with and make it a part of your daily routine.

I'd encourage you to start with a challenge. Give yourself a ten-day challenge to complete. Keep it attainable—remember minimum, target, and outrageous goals. Don't be too hard on yourself. Maybe your first goal is simply to enjoy moving every day. Give yourself permission to celebrate the small victories. Remember—you're doing this for you.

As you become more comfortable with exercise, think about starting a thirty-day challenge. Keep it simple. Don't overwhelm yourself, and don't push yourself to the point of hating it. You want to challenge yourself, but be realistic with where you are.

Don't tell yourself you're going to do fifty pushups tomorrow. First of all, if you wait until tomorrow, you probably won't do it. Start today. Give yourself a realistic goal and see if you can exceed it. Whether you hit your target or double it, it's something to be excited about!

You're likely familiar with the Nike slogan, "Just do it." Marketing slogan though it is, it's excellent advice. All the planning and prepping and thinking and waiting are only helpful at first, and then at some point you just have to do it. You will have a sense of accomplishment by getting into it, and you'll feel good about yourself. Enjoy the little wins. Give yourself a hug, a pat on the back, maybe even a gift for hitting bigger goals. You can even make a chart to track your progress with different rewards along the way!

Short Bursts

Research has proven that short bursts of exercise, even just ten minutes at a time, can be as good for your body as more prolonged periods of exercise. Even ten-minute bursts can have crazy positive effects on your immune system, heart, and body in general.

Not all workouts have to be intense. You can simply spend ten minutes dancing around the house with your spouse, which may just lead to another form of exercise. You know—the incredible passion in the bedroom that is the seductive alternative exercise of life.

The next time you feel run down, miserable, or grumpy, don't turn on the TV or grab a snack. Instead, set the alarm for ten minutes. Take a brisk walk, switch between a few of your favorite exercises, or throw on a catchy song. Watch as your short burst of exercise gets your energy up and boosts your mood. Some evidence even suggests your ten-minute intense workout can rival an hour-long session at the gym.

It's like enjoying a beautifully prepared dinner in ten minutes or whipping up a beautiful, healthy chocolate dessert. These ten-minute bursts can change your life. You can go from feeling blah to bliss in a very short period of time. It's quite incredible! In ten minutes you can clean up the kitchen. In ten minutes you can have a shower and get ready for the day. In ten minutes you can plan out your week. Or in ten minutes you can choose to change your whole entire life!

Why not take ten minutes a day for yourself and your health? It's a low investment with a huge return. Before long, those ten minutes will transform the way you feel every day.

Daily Walks

Believe it or not, going for a walk is one of the best ways to get moving.

Starting this daily habit is something wonderful—it's movement that is easy and fun and doesn't have to overwhelm your schedule. Getting outside opens up your creativity and allows your mind to declutter. When your body moves, it keeps your brain from doing too much overthinking, allowing it to focus.

You can brainstorm, imagine, daydream, and expand. Moving around lets your mind ponder, come up with ideas, organize, visualize, and just be. You'll see and notice more in the world around you. Breathe deeply, see the beauty, listen to the sounds, and take in the world. Allow yourself to find joy in the little things around you.

It takes you out of your immediate situation and reminds you of how big the world is. Walking around your neighborhood is also an excellent opportunity to meet friends, connect with your community, and encourage others with simple friendliness.

Benefits of walking also include: getting your body moving, staying agile, increasing flexibility, and helping you tone. Like most forms of exercise, it allows endorphins to enter your bloodstream, which causes an instant natural mood boost.

Just Keep Moving

Wherever you are in your fitness journey, whether you're feeling stronger by the minute or unmotivated all the time, just keep moving.

Keep going—no more stagnation, no more sedentary lifestyle for you. Your body needs to stay active, and the opportunity to do so isn't one you should take for granted.

Don't think of it as "I have to go to the gym" or "I have to go swimming." You don't have to—you get to! You are lucky to be able to run. You are blessed to have access to a gym. You have the ability to walk. Use it. Be thankful for your body and take care of it as it takes care of you. Your body will thank you.

My friend Mary is always encouraging me in this. She is dedicated to staying active and tells me how much she wants to keep playing on the floor with her grandkids. She wants to keep riding a bike and running down a trail with her family. She wants to keep walking so she can enjoy travelling and not max herself out halfway through the day. She wants to enjoy life and live the life of her dreams. She wants to live with no regrets, not missing a single opportunity.

Staying flexible, as Mary talks about, and staying in the right mindset are so important. You are young. Sixty is the new forty, and you and I have a lot more life to live and give. Movement will keep you excited about life and allow you to explore and enjoy every moment.

One of my favorite ways to keep moving is to play music while I work around the house—the kind with a strong beat that I can't help but move my hips to. Cooking dinner, cleaning the bathroom, whatever it may be—I'll step into my dancing shoes and simply have fun!

Carla and I used to love going to the lake or the river in the summer. On a hot day we'd take a tube and float out on the water. The wind would blow, and as it did, the waves moved us around. It was calm and peaceful and fun. Even if the movements weren't big or crazy, we were never still.

The water was always flowing, continually moving. This is how our bodies are meant to be—always moving with the world around us, staying agile and flexible.

Being active and flexible is a huge mental game-changer too. Exercise improves your happiness, decreases stress and anxiety dramatically, and helps you roll with the craziness of life from a more relaxed standpoint.

You might not always be in the mood, and I get this. It's still important to come from that frame of mind.

When my husband became ill with PTSD, he was housebound because of anxiety. Through this, I became stagnant. Complacent. I would tell myself I needed to stay at home and look after him, but I was making excuses. I gave up exercise. I stopped watching what I ate, consuming more and more unhealthy and processed foods. I wasn't active. It was a recipe for disaster, and before long, my health began to wane.

I was miserable, feeling more and more sorry for myself. Not much time passed before I began to get depressed myself, and my whole outlook on life spiraled downward fast.

I woke up one day and realized I'd had enough. I was frustrated with myself for neglecting my health and well-being. I knew better, and I'd allowed the circumstances to get the better of me. I had all the knowledge on how to live a happy, healthy life, but I still got side railed.

It was a lot of work to forgive myself, pick myself back up, and move forward again. I love what Les Brown says: "If you fall down and you can still look up—you can still get up!" So I did just that! I picked myself up and began to take care of myself. Movement—choosing to push forward even when I didn't feel like it gave me back myself and the love of my life.

My granddaughter is one year old. She's learning to walk and falls time after time every single day. But after each fall she picks herself up and moves forward. She's not afraid to fall because she's not failing. She learns and grows with each step. It's time we take on that attitude again, not afraid of falling, but embracing the journey.

Mary, that inspiring friend of mine, became a fitness instructor at the age of sixty. She was terrified, scared of failure, to be leading from the front. She was afraid she wouldn't remember the moves, but stepping out of her comfort zone allowed her to do more than she ever thought she could. Not only did she change her life, but she's now impacting so many others by showing women her age what they can do.

I've heard it said that "whatever you're not changing, you're choosing." Don't choose your comfort zone. Don't choose to give up on yourself.

Change your health; change your life. Before long, exercise will be the highlight of your day.

Chapter 5

Nutrition

The Sizzle

"Clean eating" is a term that's thrown around and talked about all over the place, but it's rarely defined and can seem confusing or hard to achieve. To me, clean eating could be described as a lifestyle, an ever-evolving journey. The most important thing is putting whole, real food into your body and eliminating over-processed, chemical-filled junk. You wouldn't believe how much of what we buy is really just processed crap. Instant meals, snack foods, and even basics like bread and yogurt are, more often than not, overloaded with sugar, toxins, and substances that'll do anything but add to your health. Even things like granola bars, marketed as a "healthy alternative," usually contain just as much sugar as candy bars.

Taking the time to know what you're buying, consuming, and feeding your family is an essential first step to clean eating. As you begin this process, go through your cupboards, pantry, and fridge and get rid of processed junk food. This change in your life takes a lot of commitment. Changing your eating habits (your nutrition) is a big deal and a necessary act of living a healthy and happy life.

The next time you head to the grocery store, don't allow yourself to buy any processed junk food. If you're used to buying a lot, this will be a big change. You may instinctively grab a bottle of salad dressing for dinner tonight—but realize salad dressing most definitely falls into the "processed crap" category. Instead, grab some oil and vinegar, add your own spices and whip up your own dressing! You can even go plain green if you'd rather and add extra toppings for more flavor!

After you've gotten rid of the processed junk around you, it's time to feel the sizzle. Let's be honest. We both need some sizzle and excitement in our lives, and this applies to food. At first, you might not feel any different, but after a few weeks of eating whole, clean, healthy food, your body will tell you how thrilled it is.

You'll have more energy, you'll sleep better, your immune system will be much stronger, and your mind will feel renewed and refreshed. Taking care of yourself will undoubtedly help you love yourself in a new way. You'll lose unnecessary weight naturally as you care for yourself, and your body will let you know if you eat something unhealthy. If you've never tried clean eating before, try making a game out of it. Make your first sizzle the goal and keep track of your progress to see how good you can get yourself feeling. You may have cravings for old habits, and it's important to resist those as much as you can.

Give yourself enough grace to know this isn't a test, and slipping up here or there doesn't mean you're a failure. A healthy life is a journey, and it's important to have fun with it.

You will get out what you put into it. A perfect example of that is my client Gladys. She will tell you that my Weigh Down Lifestyle program is the best thing she's ever done. When Gladys started, she went all in and didn't look back. She lost more than ten pounds in ten days right away, and this changed her life. Completely on board, Gladys felt the sizzle as soon as she got her first win. Then in the next ten days she experienced another sizzle when she was able to fit back into that gown she couldn't wear for the last four years. She could now look at herself in the mirror and say—I do feel better. I do have more energy. I feel less sluggish, and with God on my side—it is possible! She has a whole new lease on life because of making this one decision.

Today Gladys has found so many new tasty recipes within my program, and she is a living testimony to the fact that what you put into your body makes a difference. Quality in does equal quality out. She went from feeling blah to bliss in no time at all. Ahhh—the sizzle benefits.

Back to Basics

I grew up eating nutritious food. As a child, I loved being at my grandparents' farm, collecting eggs from the hen house, watching them make food entirely from scratch, and learning from their habits. Those are some of my favorite memories.

There's a practice in clean eating I like to live by called the 80/20 rule. It means to eat 80 percent clean, whole, unprocessed foods, allowing 20 percent wiggle room to treat yourself. We basically followed that on the farm, but it was entirely unconscious. We always made things from scratch because we didn't have any packaged food. Baking days were the best—coming home and biting into a fresh slice of Grandma's homemade bread or a warm cookie.

I felt the sizzle, even then. I just didn't realize it—potlucks with friends, enjoying delicious food filled with whole ingredients. We knew exactly what was in everything we were eating—and no preservatives or additives or chemicals. This was before the words genetically modified became a part of our food vocabulary.

I was blessed to grow up that way, eating clean, real food. That's not always the case today. As you embark on this journey, think about the food habits you may have established in your childhood and growing up years. What did you eat? Was it processed junk, packaged food, or made from scratch? Was it fresh fruit and garden vegetables you picked yourself?

It's important to identify the mindset and relationship you have with food to make sure you can shift appropriately if you need to. Our parents do their best, but they don't always teach us everything we need to know. And they weren't always right, even though they tried. Healthy and nutritious food may not come naturally to you—but it's so worth the lifestyle change.

Keep It Simple

Sizzle without slaving. Believe it or not, delicious, simple, and easy meals can be prepared in ten minutes or less.

If you enjoy spending time in your kitchen, then the amount of time creating meals may not matter as much to you. Sizzle in the kitchen can come with creativity as you experiment with new recipes, spices and foods you haven't tried before.

Not all of us can (or want to) take the time every day to create elaborate meals from scratch. It's a great idea to prepare some recipes on a day when you have more time, and see how long they take for future reference.

A great way to save time and money is to plan your meals and make a grocery list. You'll only have to go to the store once a week this way, and you can meal prep by batch-cooking everything you'll eat for the week. Invite your spouse or a friend to join you and spend a couple of hours cooking all you'll need! Create a different kind of sizzle in the kitchen together.

You can even stick your meals in the freezer and save yourself time in advance. If you'd rather cook fresh, try at least chopping your veggies and meat in advance so you're only in the kitchen for the actual cooking time.

Put on some music and get cooking! As I've already told you—dancing around and having fun as you get things done will not only make it more enjoyable while releasing endorphins in your brain to boost your mood, but it'll also help you feel better physically as you get active. Even in your most menopausal moments, listening to some fun tunes and preparing delicious food will make you feel alive and free.

Intermittent Fasting

In recent years, the practice of intermittent fasting has become a bit of a fad. Unlike many other popular dietary trends, fasting has been around since the beginning of time.

If you haven't tried it and want to know more about it, I highly recommend looking into it. Fasting has many scientific benefits you can read about and try for yourself. I'm not going to talk too much about this, but just know fasting has many variations. Be sure to research this at length to reap the benefits and not put yourself at risk.

Intermittent fasting is an eating regimen where you cycle between periods of eating and fasting. It doesn't specify which foods you can eat, but rather when you should eat them. There are several intermittent fasting methods, all of which split the day or week into eating periods and fasting periods.

If you want to give it a go, I suggest starting with the sixteen-to-eight-hour intermittent fasting program. You can do this quite simply—eat all your meals in an eight-hour window, and then don't eat or drink anything except water for the other sixteen hours. Many people have been successful at losing weight doing this. So you may want to have your eight-hour window (sizzle) be between nine and five, or ten and six, or do whatever works for you.

Fasting is a unique method and might be worth a trial period. It's well-loved by a large community, and trying new things will help you get to know your body and what works for you. It's okay to experiment a bit—remember, this is a journey, and you may not love everything you try. But you'll never know if you don't give it a shot. Do your research, step out of your comfort zone, and embrace the sizzle!

Supplements

Supplements are one of my favorite ways to add sizzle to my life. "Supplements" are a broad term, including everything from vitamin D capsules to essential oils.

I LOVE my oils. The scents are calming and grounding, and they help me stay energized and happy. Aromatherapy can be so soothing and is a great and easy way to find pure bliss in your life. Different oils have so many health benefits, and so much information is available on them.

A friend of mine tried oils for the first time in her water recently. She put in a single drop, having no idea it was about to change her life. She felt energized, happier, and more relaxed, almost instantly. Her senses were awakened, and she felt blissful. She fell in love immediately and has never looked back.

Essential oils are a great tool. Why not pick up a couple and try adding them to your water? You never know what might happen. Be sure to research which company you want to buy from so you are getting the right information. Essential oils have many great benefits but must be used with caution as well.

"Supplements" include a whole assortment of goodies. They can energize you and add vitality to your life. For example, a green smoothie with so many dense nutrients in one drink can make you feel like you are giving your body a boost of love, which is an essential aspect of health. Check out some of my recipes later.

Loving your body and giving it what it needs feels good. Giving your body enough water or vitamin D, letting yourself rest when it needs rest, getting moving when you need to move, enjoying the fresh air and sun, and taking care of yourself add so much sizzle to your life.

I have a friend, Peggy, who goes to Palm Springs every winter. She wants to bathe in the sun and escape the winter blues. Now that's what I call sizzle! What a way to add spice to your life.

Even just imagining a beautiful turquoise ocean, the rolling waves lapping the white sand, sitting in a lounge chair, sipping on an iced drink adds a whole lot of sizzle to my life. Did you know that imagining something can bring almost as much joy to your life as doing it?

It's true—your subconscious mind doesn't know the difference, so keep envisioning the sun's rays warming your body and give yourself some imagination sizzle. Allow your imagination to expand and become vivid in your mind and watch as your sizzle becomes real, lasting bliss.

Supplements can also be added boosts to your body through protein shakes, smoothies, moringa oleifera drinks, gogi berries, cacao bliss, and so many other wonderful superfoods that feed your body the sizzle it needs. Don't ever give up loving on yourself in this way. Something can be said for "you are what you eat"—so give yourself the quality fuel, the high octane that fuels your body the right way.

Gut Health

Believe it or not, your gut is directly connected to your brain. Countless scientific studies now show just how much what you put into your gut affects your brain and through it how you think, feel, and act.

Mental health disorders such as anxiety and depression can be either the cause or the product of gut issues. The brain is so closely tied to your digestive system that when one of them is in distress it often leads to the other.

The gut is a microbiome—a home that must be looked after with the best of care. Protect this like it's a diamond. You may have heard it said before to "love your liver" because your liver processes or filters everything you put into your body. In the same way, feeding your gut healthy products is just as important. Everything you put into your gut affects just how much sizzle you add to your life. Good things help you feel better, which will allow you to enjoy life more, which is the sizzle! It's all interconnected.

You might be asking, how do I love my gut? Well, first of all, it means giving it the right products. In this particular instance, I'm talking about foods that heal rather than damage your gut. Pre- and probiotics are absolutely vital to your health and to feeding your gut what it needs.

Prebiotics are a special form of dietary fiber that acts as a fertilizer. It feeds the friendly, good bacteria in your gut. Probiotics are live bacteria or beneficial bacteria found in certain foods or supplements like yogurt, kombucha, and other fermented foods (be sure to read the labels).

Probiotics that are similar to the ones your body makes can be taken to supplement healthy digestion. Using prebiotics and probiotics together is called microbiome therapy. You don't necessarily need to take a prebiotic, but it might make your probiotics more effective if you do.

Other ways of being kind to your gut health include habits like drinking enough water. Staying hydrated means you'll have enough liquid in your gut to allow it to digest foods easily. Believe it or not, lemons are another great source of gut health benefits. A fresh-squeezed lemon neutralizes the acids in your gut. Green tea is another easy option. If you don't already drink it, try adding it to your daily drink list or grab one next time you're out with a friend. You'll begin to love these foods and the way they make you feel.

Your gut also needs fiber. Do you even know how much fiber you're putting into your body in a day? It's time to figure out what your gut needs. Anti-inflammatory foods are great for your overall health and will help you stop feeling so bloated. Before long, you'll be feeling healthy, energetic, alive, and well. Look for the superfoods that feed your gut and see the change in the way you think, act, and feel.

Free Radicals and Antioxidants

"Free radicals" are bad toxins. They enter our bodies and try to get us feeling blue. This is not the kind of lifestyle we want. It's important to understand how much these toxins can harm us. We need to be prepared to combat their effects and fight back.

Free radicals enter your body at the cellular level. They go deep and are far-reaching. They spread throughout your body, being carried by the bloodstream. Imagine putting a rubber duck into a stream, and almost instantly the duck is far beyond your grasp. It gets carried away so quickly by the current that without realizing it you suddenly need help from a friend to get it back.

The same is true with free radicals and antioxidants. Antioxidants are our friends. They help rescue our health. They help get rid of the toxins and eliminate the harmful stuff in our bodies.

Antioxidants fight against the free radicals, but whether they can fully overpower them or not is up to you. The more antioxidants you put in your body, the better chance they will win over the free radicals. Foods with a high ORAC score (oxygen radical absorbance capacity) are foods with lots of antioxidants. If you know you have absorbed a lot of free radicals into your body, be sure to fuel your body with foods that have higher ORAC scores. Some great suggestions are broccoli, kale, dark chocolate, blueberries, acai berries, and — my personal favorite, the best one of all, a well-kept secret. It is a product I have discovered called cacao bliss, and I will share the link with you at the back of the book. You can research it later, but I wouldn't dare be without it now. Don't let the free radicals win—fight back with antioxidants and insist on taking care of yourself.

The 80/20 Rule

Despite everything I've said about nutrition and sizzle, you will always have birthdays, anniversaries, celebrations, and get-togethers where you don't want to worry about what you're eating; you're giving yourself a guilt-free day and enjoying the occasion.

This is the very reason why I love the previously mentioned 80/20 rule. Although not everyone in the clean-eating community follows this rule, I like to be flexible, willing to adapt and change. This doesn't mean I want to add a pound of sugar to my diet every day, but it might mean I'll take my granddaughters out for ice cream on a hot summer day. Or maybe if my hubby and I are out on a dinner date, we might split a piece of cheesecake.

Life is short, and I want to live it well. So I allow myself to indulge in these treats once in a while. I want to live a life of no regrets, and I never want to hear my granddaughters or husband say, "I wish you had come out for a treat with me tonight," or "Grandma . . . I wish you'd have taken me for an ice cream cone today."

Those are precious moments I refuse to give up, and those feelings of loss mean living with regrets. I want no part in that. I want to enjoy experiences, adventures, and excitement with those I love, and so I allow myself the gift of the 80/20 rule. With this rule, I decide when I will splurge. I decide when I will eat sugar. This is not a reward; this is my choosing to indulge in a treat.

It's important never to "reward" yourself with food because it leads to an unhealthy relationship with sugary snacks, and you'll want to reward yourself too often. It's better to think of a reward as a non-food item, like a bubble bath or a new pair of earrings or a walk in the park.

The key is to make the decision, enjoy the treat, and refuse to feel guilty about it. Allow yourself the pleasure at times—the key wording here is "at times." Learn to know when those times are okay, and be sure they don't sabotage all your good efforts and negatively affect your life. When you decide to indulge, then enjoy the treat.

The 80/20 rule can be used in many areas of life, not just food. Think about it as it relates to exercise or even friends—whom you hang out with for the 80/20 percent.

Sometimes it's about living dangerously, taking risks, and exploring all aspects of your life. Life truly does begin at sixty—get ready to sizzle!

Chapter 6

Relationships

One of the biggest keys to wellness is having healthy relationships. Every one of us needs people, friendships, and community. We were wired to do life with each other, and feeling alone will make it impossible to experience true bliss in your life.

Relationships, whether friendships or spousal, are essential in shaping how we see the world. We all have people who have changed our lives and helped make us who we are.

Loneliness is a feeling most of us have experienced at one time or another, and it can be crushing. Lacking in close friendships or perhaps friendships altogether can be destructive to mental health, physical health, and any chance at happiness.

Why Relationships Matter

Meeting and connecting with new people can feel uncomfortable and intimidating. It's important to remember why you're working at it and how it will enrich your life.

Even though you are working on a new, healthier, more exciting kind of life, that doesn't mean things will be perfect. We all go through things, and when life gets hard, you will need people to lean on. The relationships you build will be your support, the people you can trust and rely on. You'll show up for them, and they'll show up for you.

We all need a circle of people. Ask yourself: If I was struggling with something or in trouble, whom would I call? Are you happy with those friendships? Is your spouse someone you trust and would want to go to?

Sometimes it's not about the number of people you have in your life but about the depth and comfort of a relationship. I have casual friends I wouldn't tell my deepest secrets to, and then I have kindred spirit friends—people I trust implicitly, whom I can tell anything to and know they will be there for me, no matter what.

Having a variety of friends is also healthy and will help you grow as a person and allow you to experience more joy. Developing strong, deep friendships is a lot easier than it seems—it just takes a bit of time and dedication and a willingness to put yourself out there. Even in your marriage, restoring a foundation of friendship and emotional safety is possible. It's up to you to take the leap and make it happen.

Developing Real Friendships

Whether your phone has stopped ringing altogether, or you're hoping to deepen friendships you already have, here are some key steps to having and being a good friend.

Be Open.

Say yes to things.

We've talked a lot about your comfort zone and the risk of staying in it—and this is important when it comes to relationships too. If you only ever meet people who look the same, dress the same, and have the same interests, you may never find the kind of relationships you're looking for. You will miss an opportunity to learn about others, yourself, and the world around you.

You never know who will turn into a good friend. Some of my closest friends are very different from me, and their perspectives and experiences are incredibly enriching. Just as you would encourage a child to try different kinds of food to determine what they like, try other friendships and relationships and see which ones stick.

Be Vulnerable.

If you want to have friends you can trust, you need to show them you trust them too. Vulnerability is scary, but it's a two-way street. Without opening up in your relationships, they will stay at a surface level with no hope of going deeper. Casual acquaintances become good friends through time, laughter, and trust.

Pay Attention.

New relationships mean new people who will inevitably influence and inform you. While this is a good thing, it's important to pay attention to the ways that certain people affect you. You're chasing bliss, a life of happiness and positivity, and you don't want to be surrounded by people who will continuously bring you down and make you feel more negative. You become like the people closest to you—are they people you want to be?

Be a Good Friend First.

I can't tell you how many times I've heard people talk about feeling lonely simply because no one else was reaching out. My question to them, and you, is this: How often do you reach out to others? In order to have quality relationships, you need to show up and be a good friend first. No one will do the work for you, nor should they. You are responsible for taking charge of your life and relationships. You need to be the kind of friend to others that you want them to be for you. Not only is this fair, but it'll set the tone of your relationship on a strong note.

There are many kinds of friendships, and not everyone you meet will be a lifelong best bud. Some people come into your life for seasons and others as lessons, and some stick around for a while. It's okay to meet people you don't want to bare your soul to. Having casual friends is acceptable and an essential part of a larger circle.

Developing close relationships with even two or three people can make such a difference in your life. You will feel so much happier, safer, and enjoy life so much more.

I have a friend, Mary, who is one of the most loyal people I've ever met. I recently found out about a situation she was in a few years ago. She'd had a friend, Gloria, over visiting who suddenly felt unwell. Instead of sending her home, Mary brought her upstairs and tucked her into bed.

Little did they know, Gloria was sick with a brutal flu. Mary's husband is immuno-compromised, but Mary insisted on taking care of her friend. Gloria ended up bedridden at Mary's house for five days, during which her friend brought her food, water, and everything she needed. Despite the inconvenience of it, Mary showed up for her friend when she needed it.

That's the kind of friendship that can change your life. It's not always about agreeing on everything or getting everything right—it's about showing up for each other when it matters.

Boundaries in Friendship

As you form deep friendships, ones you want to hang on to, it's important to take care of them. Developing boundaries in friendships is an integral part of keeping them healthy. The most obvious boundary you need to establish is a strong sense of time.

How long do you want to spend with people? How long is it healthy for you to spend with your friends? Do you need more time to recharge on your own, or do you benefit from more social time?

Certain friendships and interactions may demand more energy from you, and that's okay. It's about balance, knowing your limits, and feeling free to say no when you need to.

As much as friendships and relationships are a huge part of life, they're not everything. While you're embarking on this journey, it's worth sitting down to have an honest conversation with yourself. Do you enjoy spending time with yourself? No one else can or should fill the need you have for self-satisfaction.

To love other people well, you need to love yourself first. Take time to learn this, and consider waiting to seek out other relationships until you feel confident on your own.

Marriage Relationships

When my husband and I had two young kids, he was really into fixing and working on cars. Things were going well for us. He had a steady job, the girls were the best of friends, and we were happy, for the most part.

You see, I love my family more than anything. But the girls were always running around, they had their friends, and Robert had his '69 Chevelle. He'd come home from work, feeling stressed and tired, and want to go out and work on the car. As any mother can imagine, after spending the day chasing little children, I was desperate for some kind of help or even adult conversation.

It started out casually enough, but before long he spent all his days off working on the car. I'd have to go out and plead with him to come in and spend time with our family. One day, I'd had enough. I got a sitter and told Robert we needed to go out for coffee. I sat across from him and told him I couldn't live like this anymore. I gave him an ultimatum: It's either the car—or the kids and me.

He was shocked, and it kicked him into gear. A few days later, the car was up for sale. That was never my goal, and at first I felt terrible—but Robert insisted. He knew he needed to sell it. When we got married, we knew we were committed to staying together, no matter what challenges that would bring. For better or worse, we were in it.

Marriage is many things, but easy is not one of them. Don't misunderstand me; sometimes relationships are damaged beyond repair or toxic to the detriment of either person. In those cases, you absolutely must get out. With that said, if you're hitting a hard patch, don't give up. Fight for your love, or you will lose it. To read more about our story, I have another book called *My Life with a Cop: How to Survive the Ride.*

While you're examining your relationships, don't ignore your marriage. Just because you've been together for a long time doesn't mean you don't have room to grow. Consider your relationship with your spouse and ask yourself these questions:

Is your partner someone you find easy to talk to?

Can and do you have hard conversations?

Are you truthful with each other?

Do you enjoy spending deep, meaningful time together on a regular basis?

If you see some red flags, don't panic. Relationships go through seasons, and if you're feeling some distance that means it might be time to address it.

The 5 Love Languages

An excellent tool for your marriage is a book titled *The 5 Love Languages.* Author Gary Chapman outlines the five love languages as follows: words of affirmation, quality time, receiving gifts, acts of service, and physical touch.

Each of us receives and gives love through these, but on different levels. Some of us feel most loved when our partner does things for us, meaning our top love language is acts of service. For others, verbal communication means more, or words of affirmation. Knowing this information about your spouse and even your friends makes all the difference.

It's hard to love someone well if you don't know their love languages, especially if the two of you have different love languages.

A good friend of mine spent years in her marriage feeling rejected and unloved. Physical touch was her top love language, and she didn't know how to express to her husband that the lack of it in their relationship was hurting her. It wasn't a sexual lack, but a purely affectionate habit that was missing. When she was able to explain it, he was happy to work toward adjusting his own habits to ensure she felt loved. A quick hug, holding hands on a walk, and trading back rubs were easy fixes to the problem.

The book is a great one to read together and will assuredly bring you closer together. Sometimes the best way to work on restoring your relationship is to focus most on how you can love your spouse, rather than what they're doing wrong—taking action to make them feel special and cared for, even if it's not what you most enjoy. Giving to others can bring you just as much joy, if not more, than receiving.

Emotional intimacy in your marriage is crucial. Unfortunately, it often fades away over time in relationships. Without a conscious effort to keep getting to know your spouse, sharing with them and inviting them to share, you can quickly lose the closeness you had on your wedding day.

It's a common myth that romance can fade overnight. It takes time and unwilling partners. Protecting and fighting for a healthy marriage takes effort, commitment, and a desire to truly love the other person well.

Boundaries in Marriage

Just as boundaries in friendships are important, they should be a part of your marriage as well. Believe it or not, your partner should never complete you. You shouldn't feel a need to be "fulfilled" by anyone else, even your spouse. That attitude creates an unhealthy kind of dependency that won't lead anywhere good.

As wonderful as your spouse might be, you're both human, and you will let each other down at times. When Robert was wrapped up in working on his car, I was disappointed. But if I relied on him for my feelings of value, it would have crushed me. Instead, I could ask for what I needed, and we could work on the problem. Finding your self-worth in someone else stops you from having hard conversations, and it places a burden on them that they can never carry.

My husband isn't my everything, but he is my best friend. That's the way it should be. We don't do life together because we need to, but because we get to. And even though we've had our ups and downs and challenging moments, I'd rather spend my life with him than anyone else in the world.

All relationships are complicated and hard, and nothing worthwhile comes overnight. This journey of seeking fulfilling relationships will be an adventure! An exciting opportunity to learn and grow in new ways, and being surrounded by a support system of people who love you will completely change your life. It's never too late to make a new friend, and you never know who can turn into a kindred spirit.

Chapter 7

Accountability

Why It Matters

By this point, you've begun to develop a vision for what you want your life to look like—what it will look like. Congratulations! That's a huge accomplishment and a massive step toward making it a reality. As you begin the journey of transforming your life, you're going to need to establish some accountability for yourself.

Changing your life is hard; I'd be doing you a disservice if I didn't acknowledge that. It's hard, but, wow, it is worth it! Having some accountability means you're on a team, rather than trying to cross the river on your own. I'm sure you're aware of how easy it is to fall behind on a goal if you're doing it alone.

Having an accountability partner, someone to hold you to your goals, back you up, push you when you need to be pushed, and celebrate with you will make all the difference. Adding accountability into your journey will strengthen you, motivate you, and help you to become the best version of yourself.

One of the hardest lessons to learn in my personal development journey has been that I'm not unbiased. Especially when it comes to growth in friendships and relationships, you're going to need advice and someone who is removed from the situation to call you out. You're watching life unfold through your own lens—and that's okay! But sometimes another perspective is exactly what we need to get kicked into gear and stay on the right path.

When I came up with my target weight goal, I knew I had a lot of work in front of me to get there. No matter how many times I tried to do it alone, it didn't work. I changed my diet—my lifestyle—and began exercising more than I ever had. But by myself I didn't have the motivation or support to keep going. So I got an accountability partner. I met with her every week, and she walked with me through my weigh-ins.

We kept a journal each week so I could stick to my target and my goals. It was a huge help, and I found myself more motivated and encouraged. Without that support and accountability, I don't think I would've been able to stick to my targets.

As you cross the river and go through the life changes, having someone you can talk to about it will be essential. Friends and family are wonderful, but they don't always make for great coaches. With a coach, you need someone who has already had the success you are looking for. With an accountability partner you need someone you can open up to and confide in. With both coaches and accountability partners, their goal is to help you, support you, and encourage you, and give you a kick in the butt when you need it.

What Is an Accountability Partner?

Accountability, simply put, is to be responsible to someone or something for your actions. Self-managing this is extremely difficult, if not impossible. An accountability partner is someone who is committed to helping you reach your goals. Someone you talk to consistently, who will check in and hold you responsible to yourself for the commitment you've made.

They're not there to bully you but to coach, cheerlead, and have your back no matter what. On this crazy ride, you may have moments where you need someone to hold your hand. Additionally, you will probably have moments when you need a bit of a kick in the you-know-what in order to get up and get going.

Who Is an Accountability Partner?

Remember the game Red Rover? A group of children stand in a line, holding hands, and someone tries to run through and break the hands apart. Holding hands made the line stronger. It was much harder for it to be broken when it had additional support and strength behind it. The same is true of someone who has an accountability partner.

When you feel discouraged or face challenges, being alone will make you vulnerable, and it will be harder to resist the urge to give up and go home. Being part of a team, rather than being isolated and alone, will make success much more attainable.

It's time to pick an accountability partner! During this process, you'll want to consider some key characteristics.

Can you trust this person? In order for your accountability partner to tell you the truth, you need to be able to do the same with them. Without honesty your relationship will be useless. You'll need to find someone with whom you feel comfortable being vulnerable. Can they keep your business to themselves? Will you let yourself tell them what's really going on?

Are they too close? Choosing someone like a family member or a close friend is generally not a great idea. If someone is too close to you and other people in your life, they will have a harder time being objective. Additionally, having an accountability partner who is more removed will help you feel comfortable talking to them about personal issues.

Finding a personal coach may be a great option—someone whose relationship with you is solely based on helping you grow.

What is that person's lifestyle like? While health and happiness look different for everyone, it's worth asking the question of whether or not this person lives a life you would want. If you're trying to get healthy and your accountability partner exercises once a year, that might not be your best bet. Rather, find someone who prioritizes eating well, working out, and living a balanced lifestyle. Seek out the kind of person who has achieved a level of growth to which you aspire.

In the process of launching my online business, the Weigh Down Lifestyle, my mentor was instrumental in helping me get it off the ground. This person was my business accountability coach and helped me check all my boxes quickly and efficiently. With my coach's help and my program, I've been able to see so many women transform their lives.

After my daughter Kayce had her baby, she had such a hard time losing the baby weight. She tried method after method, and nothing worked! Finally, she gave the Weigh Down Lifestyle a shot and lost more than eighty-five pounds! Not only was it a physical transformation, but a relief for her as she began to feel like herself again.

Another woman had spent more than eight hundred dollars on a weight-loss program—amongst various others—before coming to me. She'd been around the block and seen what was out there, but it was my program that finally began to work for her. She's already dropped forty pounds and is continuing to lose more.

I'm personally providing accountability calls to my clients, and one of them, Kim, has lost over twenty-five inches in the last few months. We chat once a week to check in and to help keep her accountable and ensure she's making progress. When she knows she will have to be accountable and tell me how she is doing, it makes her more apt to succeed and follow through!

Because I had a fantastic coach, one who already had the success I wanted to achieve, I am now able to give back and coach others and help them achieve their success and reach their personal goals. Their success is my driver—it's what keeps me going too!

Consistency Is Key

Having a weekly check-in with your accountability partner will ensure the effectiveness of the process and help you take responsibility for yourself. You need to take a realistic look at what you're doing—the habits, patterns, and new initiatives you're adding into your life. This helps you evaluate the ways they're adding to or taking away from your happiness.

Weekly check-ins give you a chance to celebrate your accomplishments from the past week, to tick off another box and be proud of yourself. You did it! Another week of dedicated, determined, life-changing action. Congratulate yourself and enjoy the win. Weekly check-ins also create space for feedback from you and your accountability partner.

What did you do well? What do you need to change? What's something new you'd like to try? Every week take a look at this checklist and honestly answer these questions.

Checklist

Mindset—What has your mindset been like this week? How are you talking to yourself and others? How confident do you feel, and how is your self-esteem right now?

Physical Exercise—What did exercise look like for you this week? Did you do too much, not enough, or strike a good balance? How did exercise make your body feel?

Nutrition—What did your nutrition look like this week? Did you put good, nutrient-rich food into your body? How did the food you ate affect the way you felt physically and mentally? Are you happy with your choices?

Relationships—How much time did you spend investing in relationships this week? How did it affect the way you felt? Is there anything you want to change? Did you take time for yourself this week?

Overall Well-being—Do you feel as if you're on track with where you want to be? Be truthful and honest with yourself. Allow yourself room for growth. You need to allow for setbacks. It's a marathon, not a sprint. Your goal here is to keep moving forward. This is your life. Two steps forward and one step back are still ahead. So kudos to you for being brave enough to step across this river with me.

What have you learned so far?

I want to congratulate you for picking up this book in the first place. I'm super proud of you for being willing and ready to admit you need to change and for loving yourself enough to know you deserve more. You've made so much progress already; don't you dare give up now. Pat yourself on the back and take a minute to celebrate what you're doing for yourself.

After making the decision to cross this river, you made a plan. Your plan is working. We worked on your mindset because without a mental shift you won't shift anywhere else. We explored exercise and learned about the importance of moving your body every day. We've explored nutrition and how what you put into your body affects your overall wellness.

Discussing relationships brought up boundaries, letting go, and learning to love ourselves as well as other people. Accountability, as we just talked about, is the key to implementing lasting change in all these areas.

Now we're at a point where we have to do some dirty work. We need to explore the past and what regrets we may be holding on to. We're almost done! We are making good progress, with even better things ahead. Stay with me!

We've come too far; we can't turn back now. It's time to fix our eyes on the future, on the life we're dreaming of, and keep fighting until every bit of it is ours.

Chapter 8

Life without Regrets

You are almost there—across the river, that is. Just one step away. You've made so much progress. Look over your shoulder, just for a moment, to see your old self back on the riverbank. You may feel sad, seeing the lonely, miserable person you used to be. She looks like a wilted flower—stooped over—ready to give up. She isn't someone you want to be.

It's okay to feel sad for who you used to be—but don't stay in it. You now have a valuable set of tools to live the life you want. You are ready to try new things—someone who is passionate about life again. You're ready to stop feeling stuck and celebrate life, to do something wild and crazy that exhilarates you and fills you with joy.

This is an exciting and historical time in your life, and it's one worth enjoying. Life is too short not to get excited. As we approach this last step, don't be afraid to dream big.

The goal here is to live a life with no regrets, so be honest with yourself about what you want out of life.

Your Passion

Take out a piece of paper and a pen and ask yourself this question: What do you truly want to do before you die? This isn't morbid thinking, but intentional living. It's deciding what is important to you. Make a list of at least ten things right now that you know you want to do.

The biggest regrets people have are not things they did, but things they didn't do. That's why it's important to identify what you don't want to miss. Have you been dying to travel somewhere special? Do you want to go on a special date with your spouse? Spend more time with your grandkids? Find the love of your life?

Whether it's leaving an inheritance for someone special, swimming with dolphins, trying a particular food, or taking grandkids on a trip, whatever is important to you, write it down. Identify your ten big desires. You've done so much work in your life and on yourself; you deserve to fulfill them. For your life to begin now, you must be brave enough to take it back. That means fighting for what you want.

All of us are passionate about one thing or another. It's time to explore it, enjoy it, and be happy. Oliver Wendell Holmes Sr. said this: "Many people die with their music still in them. Too often it is because they are always getting ready to live. Before they know it, time runs out."

Don't spend your life waiting for it to start—actually LIVE! It's a beautiful thing to be passionate about something, but life only happens when you take action. Not just breathing and existing, but chasing the things you care about. Leave your legacy with your music played loud.

If you're having trouble rekindling passions and getting overly enthusiastic, make a commitment to try something new every week—a new form of exercise, an art class, a new city, a new book, or a different coffee shop. Introduce new experiences into your life and, if something thrills you, chase after it for all it's worth.

A friend of mine went to a concert where the Nylons were performing. The Nylons were an acapella group, most known for the classic song "The Lion Sleeps Tonight." After the concert my friend told me she could have sat and listened to them sing for hours and hours. Her exact words were that they had "energized the life out of her." What an experience—and a worthy goal for how to live every single day! With the life energized right out of you.

Embrace your passion. Let it fill you up and be the driving force behind everything you do. At this point in your life, nothing should be meaningless. Every lesson you've learned in this book should be implemented with a passion and desire to live a healthy life.

Your Purpose

By now I hope you know that your life truly can begin at sixty. Today! I hope you see your passion and are ready to share it with the world. You've always had a purpose, but now you feel it. Now you want to shout it from the rooftops! No longer dragging your feet, you want to get out of bed in the morning. You can see yourself bounding out of bed, excited to start your day because you have so much to offer the world.

Once upon a time, you were a little girl with dreams and the world was your playground. You used to run wild and free; and somehow the cares of the world began to steal your heart, and your imagination turned grey. Your bubbles popped, and you stopped believing in magic. But as you slept that white horse and the charming prince came in one night and blew some pixie dust over you. Finally, when you awoke, you felt as if you were plugged in. You lay there and began to imagine—to dream. For the first time in years, you allowed your mind to take you to never-never land. You saw the prince get the girl, the dragon slain, and the princess saving the village.

What village needs saving in your world? Which woman around you needs your recipe for joy? What mission do you know is yours to fulfill before your life is over? Is there a story you need to tell?

If you know you have a mission and a purpose inside your heart that's about to explode if you don't tell someone,

I want to encourage you right now—please tell ME! I would love for you to private message me or go to my Facebook page and let me know how this book has changed your life. I want to hear about how you went from lonely and blue to having found joy and purpose in your life again. I want to hear your story about how the grass became green once again for you. I'd love to hear about how your imagination took you to a faraway place or about how you saw your "sign" in the sky.

You know your story, and you know some people will resonate with you—so don't waste a moment. Go out with passion and purpose and write your own recipes. If you must, start with the bare bones and add the spice later. Whatever you do, just begin. Will your recipe be an adventure? A charity? A vacation with your grandkids? Writing a book? It's all up to you—your life begins at sixty too—NOW!

Your Pursuit

Now that your life has begun and you're ready to live it, you need to ask yourself one more question. What is your pursuit?

What's the next step for you? What do you want to chase after, to add to your life? I often hear the words from women who are on this journey: "I want to be FREE." As I always say, you need to identify what you want to be free from—debt, danger, anger, self-doubt, excess weight, negative people? Do you need freedom from procrastination, stress, poor eating habits?

Maybe you need freedom from a toxic friendship or relationship or feeling the need to please other people. You know now that life is more than just running out the clock. You're ready to take back your life, so don't you dare stop now. You've made the choice to change. You've got the tools, the plan, the accountability, the mission—so JUMP!

You've done so much already—you've crossed the river and overcome the fear that was holding you back. You've figured out what you're afraid of and stepped out of your comfort zone. You have broken the chains around your limbs.

A few months ago, my coach gave me a valuable lesson. A simple statement, but it ended up being one of the biggest "aha" moments of my life. "The greater the barrier, the greater the success." It hit me hard because it's so very true. The harder you must work for something, the more you fight for it, the sweeter it is when you have it. Not everything is worth fighting for, but your happiness most certainly is. And when you've earned it yourself, it feels so very wonderful.

What are your barriers, and how have you gotten past them? Have you had a huge wall to get over? If so, how high was the wall? How did you get over it?

Take the time to remember this journey, the celebrations and the struggles. Did someone lift you up to the top of your barrier? Did you get a chair to stand on, a ladder, or dig a tunnel right underneath it? Do you feel the difference now, having made it to the other side?

You are an overcomer. You have made it through challenge after challenge and are free to embrace a life of happiness. There is a celebration waiting for you, and it's going to be a party. You have the tools at your fingertips now, and you can do it quickly and joyfully, dancing your way to the finished product. Your goals will give you passion and a reason to get up and keep going. You will love yourself because you are taking care of yourself and leaving a legacy—your future is waiting for you, and life is about to begin.

Remember your starting goal? The life you barely dared to dream of? Picture it now—see it in color. Think of the things you currently have that seemed impossible previously. While you are thinking of these, now make them ten times bigger. Watch the colors get brighter, more vivid. Take time to soak it up, to picture how much further you can go. How bright and wonderful the world is, and now you know it in a whole new way. Don't stop now. Keep going for it.

Life Begins at 60! Life begins today, whatever age you are. You will find so many recipes for joy, and you get to pick the recipe you are starting with today. You are free to fly into your pursuit of happiness.

Chapter 9

The Other Side

Where You've Been

Think of a time when you felt powerless. Maybe as a child, when you tried to use your voice and no one listened to you. Perhaps as a young adult, you experienced just how cruel life can be and realized you couldn't do anything.

Maybe it was when you began this book, when your life was far from where you wanted it to be, and you weren't sure if things would ever change.

Take a moment here to reflect on all you've accomplished. You are amazing. You knew you wanted more out of life, and you fought for it. You refused to settle for a life that was less than what it could be and chose to become a better, kinder, happier, healthier you—a truer version of yourself.

I want to congratulate you. You just crossed a huge river and completed some difficult steps, and you didn't fall in. Even when things got rough, you didn't give up. Thank you for trusting me, for trusting yourself, and for taking the first step.

That first step into the rest of your life signaled you were sick and tired of living in mediocrity or maybe even misery. You were ready for more. You envisioned what life could be, dared to dream and hope for the things you never thought you could have in your life.

Then you made a plan. You didn't stop with wishful thinking but took action. You set goals, figured out exactly what you needed to do to get from point A to point B, and worked for it. Pushing yourself physically, to get in better shape, to maximize the energy, joy, and potential in your life was hard—but you kept moving forward.

You've stepped out of your comfort zone and tried new things. You've met new people; become bolder and stronger; and overcome fear and self-consciousness that was defeating you.

You matter, and you deserve love—and by now, you're starting to feel that for the first time in a long time. You know you matter. Believing in yourself didn't feel natural, but you now know you have something to give back to humanity. You have a purpose, and you climbed over the wall. That barrier was big—huge, in fact; but if you hadn't climbed over you'd still be on the other side of the bank, slumped over, your soul slowly dying.

Now you are alive and thriving, and life is just beginning. This is going to be the best phase of your life, and you feel ready to rock. Your masterpiece has begun.

Here is where you need to take out your pencil and draw on your own. No one else can tell you what it should look like, but a legacy starts to form as it takes shape. From your own hand, you draw a wonderland around you. The only limit is your imagination, and it's up to you how far you can go.

You are a brilliant, amazing individual, created with a purpose, and you have an important role to play in this world.

What's Next?

The blood, sweat, and tears you've put into this journey are not in vain. Furthermore, the journey isn't over. Life begins at sixty, remember?

By now, you know that working on yourself, creating a better life, is hard but worth it. You know the feeling of accomplishment that comes when you hit a target and see the change in yourself. As you celebrate your progress, don't lose sight of your vision for the rest of your life.

Don't let your new habits become New Year's resolutions that only last a couple of weeks. Stick with them! Hang onto your accountability partner and continue to seek out new friendships, depth in relationships, and a happier, healthier lifestyle.

If weight loss is one of your main goals, I can help. Check out my program "The Weigh Down Lifestyle," designed to help you keep transforming your life to become the happiest, healthiest you. There'll be more information at the back of the book, and I promise you, you won't regret it. I've seen so many women finally achieve what they've been working for through this program, and it's a beautiful thing.

Now that you know to keep moving forward, you need to practice saying yes to new opportunities. As you practice self-love, don't ever refuse an opportunity to better or grow yourself. Challenging opportunities are the ones that shape you and change you the most, and you'll never know what you're capable of until you try.

Let me tell you about a woman who wanted to be a speaker. She had the dream and the passion but thought she had no story to tell. She took the first step across the river and imagined herself on speaking stages. Each day as she woke up, she saw herself in front of a crowd. She continued this visualization process day after day, and before long an opportunity presented itself to her. She took the next step and said yes.

What happened next was amazing. Once she said yes to the first thing, miracles appeared. She went to a seminar and met remarkable new people. She learned and grew. She dug deep. Like the tree, she was planted by the river, and her roots went down deep and spread out. She found a team, and together they grew.

Say yes to everything you can. Do not turn down an opportunity. Say yes, but give yourself the freedom to fall. Remember, falling isn't a failure; it is just another learning opportunity.

You will probably fall and scrape your knees a couple of times. That's okay—in fact, it's encouraged. Never letting yourself fall means you're never jumping, and if you don't jump, you can't fly. Self-made limitations are the hardest ones to throw off, so make sure you're not letting them stop you. If you feel as if you're starting to self-sabotage, sit down and write down—and speak out loud—the things you're telling yourself about who you are. Sometimes, being honest about what you're feeling will show you how silly it is.

One of the best things you can do with this gift, this second chance you've made for yourself, is to share it. Too many women feel this way, run down and miserable in their sixties, living their most depressed lives instead of their best ones. Whom do you know you can encourage? Whom can you invite to grab coffee? Whom can you tell about this extraordinary transformation in your life?

You were born for greatness, designed to thrive, and built for strength. Don't look back with sadness at who you were, and don't stay stuck in the what-ifs of life. Embrace gratitude for where your journey has brought you and every scar it's given you because it made you who you are: beautiful, kind, compassionate, and a strong, powerful force to be reckoned with.

You are on the cusp of your future, and you are in charge of where it goes. This is your ship to sail. Pursue growth, happiness, and a full life. Keep dreaming, working, and believing for more.

Your life is just beginning.

Conclusion

The Weigh Down Lifestyle—What Is It?

You know how so many women have trouble losing weight? Well, my passion is to help women lose weight without being on a diet, even if they have tried before and failed. You haven't failed dieting. Dieting has failed you!

God gave me a vision and a purpose many years ago. God gave me a passion for health, fitness, and wellness, and He also gave me a desire to motivate and encourage women. I want to enjoy living a happy, healthy life, to be the best version of me, and I know that other women feel the same way. I believe being a healthy weight is a vital piece of the puzzle—it's crucial to being the best I can be.

The Weigh Down Lifestyle community is a place where Christian women all over North America are coming together and uniting—transforming their lives by fueling their bodies with the right foods ten days at a time. I believe Quality In = Quality Out.

I love the analogy of a vehicle. When you go to the service station to fuel your gasoline engine, what do you put in the fuel tank? Gasoline or diesel? You might think this is a silly question, but if you were to put diesel into your gas-powered car, what do you think would happen? RIGHT! It would break down, and it might even blow up! But, for sure, it would not run well.

It's the same with your body. When you put the right fuel, the right nutrient-dense foods in your body, it works well. The right fuel is the whole, healthy foods God gave us to enjoy—not the processed junk the media culture and the fad diets have led us to believe is healthy. Eating whole foods in their most natural state or form and making food from scratch is what I'm referring to here. It has to do with cutting out the chemicals, the preservatives, the artificial flavors and sweeteners, as well as the sugars and highly processed foods that are causing disease and causing us harm.

Remember my client Gladys, who said she had tried every diet out there? She had given up and was devastated with her life. She even spent more than eight hundred dollars on a weight-loss program she didn't follow through with—that is until she found the 10-Day Weigh Down program. She said, "Ruth's 10-Day Weigh Down program has transformed my life. I thank God for finding Ruth and her program at just the right time. This has given me my life back, and I am loving my healthy lifestyle now, with

God at the center." These types of testimonials keep me motivated and inspired to carry on with my mission. They are what drives me!

The 10-Day Weigh Down program is exactly that. It's ten days of following a nutrient-dense meal plan that allows your body to heal itself from the inside out. It's a program that is designed to help you kick start your body into healing mode—to eat clean and healthy for ten days in a row and neutralize your cravings so you can stop going back to that junk food cupboard!

My 10-10-10 Plan Works!

In ten days you will feel the difference.

In another ten days you will see the difference.

And in another ten days—so thirty days from now—you will hear the difference.

It's short and doable, a simple plan that works; it's a new way for women to achieve their first WIN in just ten days. It's amazing because it WORKS. You can do anything for ten days. It's short for a reason, because psychologically when you achieve your first win you have faith in yourself for the very first time. It is doable, and you begin to believe in yourself—something you haven't done in a very long time.

With this program you will experience a transformation in your weight loss and your way of thinking; you will have a mindset shift and gain more confidence in yourself.

Because of a beta test I did with a hundred women, women of every shape and in every phase of life, I know this plan works. Every woman who followed the plan lost weight.

With the 10-Day Weigh Down program, you will receive ten days of encouragement videos from me. You will also get ten days of e-mails from me to motivate you each day. You will have psychological techniques to use to remove the fear, doubt, and limiting beliefs that creep into your mind to bring you down. You will move daily and meet other beautiful women doing the same journey as you. You will NOT be alone because being alone doesn't work. We are designed for fellowship, and these beautiful souls will become more than friends. They will spur you on to reach your own goals, and together we can achieve tremendous success.

Follow me in my journey and let's live a happy, healthy life together, with God at the center. Join my Weigh Down Lifestyle community today.

Testimonials

I love Ruth Verbree's program of clean eating, with many delicious recipes to choose from. I love the fact that Ruth inspires us with the Word of the Day (WOD) and a Bible devotional as well as Facebook encouragements, where we can also encourage each other. I lost over twenty-five inches and am continuing to maintain my weight loss with the Weekly Accountability Calls (WAC). Thanks, Ruth, for faithfully creating a program for us that really works!

Kim Alviano

Losing weight, reducing inflammation, sleeping better, reduced heartburn, and improved GERD are just a few of the results I have had while doing the 10-Day Weigh Down challenge! Ruth and her team provide a Christian community program that encourages us to bring God into the journey. This component, along with the fully proportioned delicious recipes, makes this program a lifestyle eating plan anyone can follow. Thanks, Ruth Verbree, for all your hard work and dedication and, most important, for listening to the call God has placed on your life to help women realize we are chosen for greatness by God! And with God in the journey, we will succeed!

Sharon Hausch

I have been with Ruth almost from the beginning. I love her program. I have tried many other diets that work for a short time, but then the weight comes back on as soon as I stop the diet. Ruth's program is not a diet but a lifestyle change! It's about learning to treat your body like the temple it should be. There is no counting calories or points or carbs and no weighing every morsel. This program is about learning to eat healthy and clean. The support from Ruth and her team is amazing. The food is delicious, and the recipes are easy to prepare. The best part is that it really WORKS! I would recommend this program to anyone. Try it—you won't be disappointed. The only thing you will lose is the weight!

Teen Bickford

I was blessed to find Ruth's program online during the height of the covid crisis. I had been gaining weight and feeling horrid and depressed. Ruth and Kayce are remarkable, motivated and enthusiastic. With their support I have lost twenty-two pounds and counting!

Paula Daniels

I am so blessed to have discovered this AMAZING program! Ruth provides terrific support, advice, and great results. Try it, and you won't be disappointed. You will love it as much as we do!

Goska Kadlubicki

I am so blessed to have found Ruth's program on Facebook. I had gained weight, wasn't happy with myself, and wasn't able to walk much. Ruth and her team are so amazing and motivating. I started the program, and in approximately three months I have lost over thirty pounds, and I'm still counting. I am feeling great, and I'm now also walking again. Plus, the recipes are amazing.

Patsy Randell

I love this program. I'm fifty-eight, hitting sixty soon, and I want to be the best version of me.

Mary Bartholomew

I'm so grateful to God that I found Ruth's 10-Day Weigh Down challenge. I lost more than thirty-six pounds in just over two months! And my husband is down almost twenty pounds! We are feeling better than we have in years! I'm so thankful for this group and this new lifestyle.

Julie Allard

I always paid large amounts for weight-loss programs I didn't follow through with. I've even spent more than eight hundred dollars on a weight-loss program I didn't complete. That is until I found Ruth's program! The foods are amazing. I lost 10.1 pounds in the first ten days! Wow! I am so overwhelmed with joy. Thanks be to God, Ruth Verbree, and all the women who are part of this platform. You got this. God's got you. Keep going, and you will see results.

Gladys Akuoko

I am so happy I found this Weigh Down Lifestyle! I feel so much better about eating the right food and the right portions. I have lost weight and am not hungry, and I don't have cravings for sugary foods any longer! Ruth gives us so much support, and I love that our values align as she is a Christian. It works when God is involved!

Donna Michaelson

I first saw Ruth Verbree in an interview when she spoke about mental health, and I knew then that Ruth was a person I wanted to learn from. In 2020 I joined her online lifestyle program with a goal to lose weight. What I found, though, was that Ruth's programs involve so much more; they include the physical aspect of weight loss and an encouraging intertwined circle of physical, mental, emotional, intellectual, spiritual, and social well-being. Ruth's warmth has built an ever-increasing group of "Women Chosen for

Greatness." The women in this community express and share their own personal benefits of her online programs on her regular coaching sessions. Thank you, Ruth Verbree, for being you and sharing what living your life on purpose looks like. Thank you for sharing how this has impacted you and your family and how I (we) can translate this to mine (ours).

Nadira Dyalsingh

I found Ruth Verbree and her program at just the right time. I was depressed and discouraged in my life. I had no support, and I was doing it alone. Ruth really is an amazing lady who has so much energy and encouragement to give. She is so full of information on health and fitness. I have never had much support growing up my entire life, and I feel very blessed to have met Ruth to have hope and support. Ruth's encouragement and coaching calls are continuously helping me lose weight, learn to love myself again and finally take care of myself. I thank God that I found Ruth and her team at the perfect time, and her program is transforming my life one step at a time.

Jolyn Loucks

About the Author

Ruth Verbree knows she is a Woman Chosen for Greatness. She has been blessed to have had some incredible life experiences that have led her to where she is today. Ruth decided 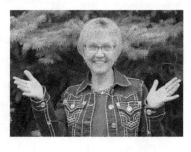 early in her marriage to follow her husband in his career. In this journey that lasted more than thirty-five years, Ruth had many different job opportunities in different cities, but the job she loved the most and was very passionate about was owning her own gym for women. It was there her passion for helping women through faith and fitness was born and truly ignited.

With each transfer her husband took, Ruth gave up her job to follow her husband. After retirement, Ruth and her husband, Robert, were so looking forward to the best time of their lives together. But then tragedy struck. Instead of travelling the world and enjoying some much-needed downtime together, Ruth became the caregiver to her husband, who fell victim to PTSD (post-traumatic stress disorder) and almost committed suicide. This journey found her spiraling downward herself, and she became very aware that if she didn't soon take care of herself she would not be able to care for her loved ones around her. This awareness changed the trajectory of their lives.

This journey propelled Ruth forward to attend several seminars and take personal development courses. Ruth has now become an award-winning author and an international speaker on mental wellness, and through this she realized she had purpose in her life again.

This opened up a whole new online world for Ruth, where she realized she could once again fulfill her dream of helping women as she had before, to lose weight and learn to love themselves again. This time, though, she decided to narrow her audience and focus on Christian women. Ruth recognized a genuine need for being real, for an outpouring of encouragement, love, and motivation for Christian women to know they were worthwhile and deserved to live a happy, healthy life. This included being a healthy weight as well.

Ruth now has an online private Facebook community where she leads and guides Christian women through her

Weigh Down Lifestyle program. Her clients often hear her say about the Weigh Down Lifestyle:

In ten days, you will FEEL the difference;

In twenty days, you will SEE the difference;

In thirty days, you will HEAR the difference!

Ruth is very passionate about helping her clients lose weight without being on a diet, even if they had tried before and failed. Ruth helps women learn to love themselves again, embrace life, and live a life with no regrets.

You will hear Ruth say, "I believe life begins at sixty! I also believe life begins for you today, whatever age you are! So take action and start living your happy, healthy life today. If not now, when?"

Additional Resources

https://www.weighdownlifestyle.com

Products I love:

Cacao Bliss. This is an awesome guilt-free product that makes me happy. http://rverbree.dmsupps.hop. clickbank.net/?pid=cacaoaffiliate&tid=

Young Living. Essential oils are a part of my everyday routine. https://www.youngliving.com/vo/#/signup/ne wstart?sponsorid=23431267&enrollerid=23431267&i socountrycode=CA&culture=en-CA&type=member

Asili Protein shakes. My favorite protein powder for smoothies. https://ruthverbree.myasiliglobal.com

Endnotes

1 https://www.healthywomen.org/your-health/
menopause-aging-well/will-your-marriage-survive-
menopause

2 https://www.ourbodiesourselves.org/2013/10/what-
percentage-of-women-are-satisfied-with-their-body-
image-survey-says/#:~:text=But%20a%20new%20
study%20published,satisfied%20with%20their%20
body%20size.&text=Participants%20were%20
overwhelmingly%20white%20

3 Luke 6:31, New International Version

4 Proverbs 23:7, New King James Version

5 Mathew 6:25-27, New International Version

6 Raymond Aaron, Orbit Coach

A free ebook edition
is available with the
purchase of this book.

To claim your free ebook edition:

1. Visit MorganJamesBOGO.com
2. Sign your name CLEARLY in the space
3. Complete the form and submit a photo of the entire copyright page
4. You or your friend can download the ebook to your preferred device

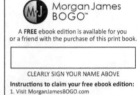

Morgan James
BOGO™

A **FREE** ebook edition is available for you or a friend with the purchase of this print book.

CLEARLY SIGN YOUR NAME ABOVE

Instructions to claim your free ebook edition:
1. Visit MorganJamesBOGO.com
2. Sign your name CLEARLY in the space above
3. Complete the form and submit a photo of this entire page
4. You or your friend can download the ebook to your preferred device

Print & Digital Together Forever.

Snap a photo   Free ebook   Read anywhere

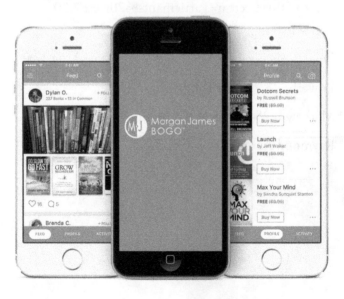

CPSIA information can be obtained
at www.ICGtesting.com
Printed in the USA
JSHW041429060821
17641JS00002B/119